DEAR LUISE

Dorrit Cato Christensen

DEAR LUISE

A story of power and powerlessness
in Denmark's psychiatric care system

Translated from the Danish
by Peter Stansill

Foreword by Poul Nyrup Rasmussen,
former Danish Prime Minister and
Member of the European Parliament

JORVIK

Jorvik Press
Portland, Oregon

Formatting: Keith Carlson

ISBN-13: 978-0988412200

ISBN-10: 0988412209

Original Danish edition published in Copenhagen
by Løfbergs Forlag, 2011

First U.S. edition, 2012

JORVIK PRESS
PMB 424, 5331 SW Macadam Ave., Suite 258
Portland, Oregon 97239-3871, USA

About the Author

Dorrit Cato Christensen is a retired teacher living in Copenhagen, Denmark, who devotes her time to advocating for better treatment of the mentally ill.

She is president of *Død i Psykiatrien* (Death in Psychiatric Care), a Danish support organization for families and friends of patients who have died from overmedication and for those concerned about the well-being of loved ones undergoing medication-based psychiatric treatment.

She is also active in several European organizations with similar goals, including the European Union's Agency for Fundamental Rights.

Acknowledgements

Quotations on page 9 and 131 are from *Asperger's Syndrome: A Guide for Parents and Professionals* by Tony Attwood; Jessica Kingsley Publishing, first edition (London 1998), pages 179 and 184. Copyright © Tony Attwood 1998.

Quotations on pages 57 and 63 are from *Modernity and the Holocaust* by Zygmunt Bauman, Polity Press (Cambridge, UK) 1989, pages 103 and 159. Copyright © Zygmunt Bauman 1989.

Quotations on pages 36, 84 and 176 are from *The Little Prince* by Antoine de St.-Exupéry, translated from the French by Katherine Woods, Egmont (London) 2009, pages 33, 44 and 68. Copyright © Editions Gallimard (Paris) 1946 and 2009.

CONTENTS

Foreword... i

Preface..iv

1. July 15, 2005 1

2. April 29, 2002 3

3. I am not mentally ill... 9

4. Childhood in Brumleby...................................... 20

5. Kindergarten... 25

6. Scene change... 28

7. Starting school... 32

8. Afterschool center 36

9. Deterioration 41

10. Neurology Department 45

11. Child psychiatry ward 49

12. If I had a million 55

13. The condition worsens 57

14. 'Best' treatment home... 63

15. Epilepsy: wrong diagnosis................................... 72

16. Doing my best as a mother? 80

17. Documents pile up.. 84

18. Hope wanes... 89

19. Epilepsy hospital 96

20. A turning point 99

21. 'Help' from Social Services.................................... 104

22. New label: 'schizophrenic'................................... 111

23. National Hospital... 117

24. Coercion doesn't work... 125

25. Free from hallucination.. 129

26. Drugs and hallucinations 136

27. Paranoid schizophrenia....................................... 143

28. Committed for treatment 148

29. A five-minute consultation................................... 152

30. More of the same.. 159

31. A storm of accusations 166

32. Coercion and reprisals.. 169

33. Return to hell.. 176

34. Even more medication... 180

35. Commotion in the ward 185

36. Disempowerment... 192

37. Destiny calls... 197

38. 'An unintended event'... 202

Epilogue: Fighting the system.................................... 207

Foreword

'Mom, won't you tell the world how we're treated?' This was Luise's last request to her mother, Dorrit Cato Christensen. She wanted her to describe the treatment she had received in the Danish mental health care system. With this book Dorrit fulfills her daughter's wish.

What follows is a heartrending account of a life in our psychiatric care system, a life cut tragically short – the same fate suffered by many vulnerable people being treated for mental health problems. Every year more at-risk psychiatric patients end up like Luise – we know that this population's lifespan averages 15 to 20 years less than others in their age group. This is a clear sign that we have to change the way we treat psychiatric patients.

We must improve conditions by offering quality time, attentiveness, compassion, evenhandedness and respect to every patient, so we can design the best treatment solution for each person. We need to talk openly about mental health issues and strengthen our networks of patients, families and friends. To this end I have set up a virtual meeting place, the website Psykisksaarbar.dk, now consulted by a growing population in Denmark. In 2009 I took the initiative to found an association called Det Sociale Netværk af 2009 (The Social Network of 2009), bringing together a wide range of national voluntary mental health organizations in a joint effort to improve conditions in Denmark for the mentally ill and their relatives. The organization of which Dorrit Cato Christensen is president, Død i Psykiatrien (Death in Psychiatric Treatment), is now part of our network.

I come in contact with many people who have been, or currently are, admitted to a psychiatric ward. Most have inside experience of various facilities and all agree that there are significant differences in approach from one institution to the next. A young girl said to me: 'As soon as you set foot in the ward you know what kind of hospital stay you're in for.

Whether the mind-set is caring and responsive, or whether the place is ruled by coercion, constant evaluation and a staff that ignores you.'

We should not, in all conscience, allow sub-standard treatment in a country like Denmark, yet it happens all the time. I have often heard patients say: 'You must be strong to be psychologically vulnerable.' When studies show that psychiatric caregivers harbor more negative expectations and prejudices about the mentally vulnerable than the general population, it means there is a problem inherent in our mental health care system. This is exacerbated by a dreadful lack of resources in psychiatric treatment wards.

The most important thing to remember is that first and foremost we are all human beings. We must not forget this for one second, before any incapacity or vulnerability is analyzed, defined and written down. This is why it is so important to see behind the facade of a diagnosis. A diagnosis is like an overcoat – the real person is found underneath it. This is one part of her daughter's life story that Dorrit describes so movingly for us – her personhood, her humor, her compassion and her zest for life.

When I meet people who support The Social Network, who form networks on our website Psykisksårbar.dk, or participate in our regular Sunday get-togethers, it strikes me how similar we humans really are and how much we have in common. There is basically no real difference between you and me and a person who happens to have been given a psychiatric diagnosis. It is not a question of these people being completely different, but more that sometimes they may experience so much inner noise that they are thrown off-balance and become vulnerable.

The most important thing we can do for psychiatric patients is not to keep them isolated. Loneliness is their worst enemy. And it is crucial that we nurture hope, that we hope and believe we can find the best in each other, and that we make room for the individual. Hope is the vital life-giving elixir for the soul, mind and body – to be able to sense that the people around you believe in you, that you are valued, that you are needed. We become whole when others believe in us. And we're most likely to find this when we feel the solidarity of good fellowship.

I would like to thank Dorrit Cato Christensen for her work with mental health patients and their families and friends, and for the very important work she is doing as president of the association Død i Psykiatrien. Her book is a poignant contribution to the debate, in which she openly and candidly tells the story of her daughter's sad fate and gives us a glimpse of our mental health care system groping for the right treatment. Luise's hospital records show that she told her caregivers she felt she could not tolerate the drug treatment they prescribed and wanted them to phase it out. But instead of less medication, she got more. This turned out to be fatal.

Many patients and relatives will already be familiar with the situations and events Dorrit portrays here. Many will see their own lives reflected in this story and perhaps even find the energy to fight for a dignified life. I also hope that mental health practitioners will read the book, then stop and think carefully about how they can deepen their professional skills through respect for the individual. We can be certain of one thing – pills are not and never will be enough. We must constantly listen to our patients and think carefully about whether we are giving the right medicine to the right person. The 'medicine' that always works for the psychologically vulnerable is to approach them with compassion, nurturing, trust and calmness.

Poul Nyrup Rasmussen
Danish Prime Minister 1993-2001
Member of European Parliament 2004-2009

PREFACE

This book is about my beloved daughter Luise, who died tragically in 2005 from overmedication while being treated in the Danish mental health system. Her untimely death received wide media coverage, which prompted other people to come forward with similar stories.

In recent years I have been active in the public debate on this subject, in associations formed by families and friends of victims, and as a member of Copenhagen City Council's discussion group on psychiatric issues. Through these interactions I have learned of many other tragic fates – evidence that Luise's sorrowful history is far from unique.

For years I have systematically written everything down, so I can provide exact dates and content from meetings and conversations, though there are several medical chart entries referenced here that I first became aware of after Luise's death.

My goal is to draw attention to the many patients diagnosed as schizophrenic who, like Luise, drag themselves through life in the 'neuroleptic straitjacket' of heavy medication. This treatment can produce irreversible side-effects and, at worst, lead to death. Such patients are a mere shadow group that appears in statistics under the category of 'chronic schizophrenics.' These sufferers are often left to their own devices and are paid little mind by either case workers or politicians. We need to take a serious look at the treatment they receive.

I am not against treatment with psychoactive drugs, I am simply trying to raise awareness of how destructive psychiatric treatment can become when it is poorly regulated, neglects timely care standards, and when the patient is viewed as a mere diagnostic case rather than a person with resources.

It was hard for me to witness what I saw as the wrong treatment for Luise and still not be heard by the people responsible. So in desperation

I started to write. The following lines are the introduction to the book I started to write to Luise in 2002, three years before she died:

Dear Luise. Once that strong antipsychotic medicine wears off, I hope we can sit and talk about what I've written down and that you might add your important comments on how you've experienced the many years you've spent in the mental health care system...

At that point I had no idea how bad things would get, and that Luise would never read a word of what I'd started to write. I still want to disseminate what I originally wrote. But since the most important element – Luise's own words – is missing, I have had to change much of the original formulation.

I shall do my utmost to faithfully reflect Luise's feelings and thoughts in what was planned as a sort of conversation between Luise and me but which has now become a document about Luise written by me. Luise herself never got the chance to contribute.

This is a highly personal, painful story about my darling daughter with the beautiful mind, but the reports I include on the Danish treatment system apply to a very large group of mentally ill patients who are subject to the same inhuman treatment as Luise. For them, disempowerment, overmedication, and coercion – especially veiled coercion – are a big part of everyday life.

This is about a treatment system that doesn't see the mentally ill as human beings but as diagnoses.

It is about all the families and friends who wage a sad and hopeless struggle to get a decent quality of life for a loved one.

Luise often asked me: 'Mom, can't you tell the world how we're being treated?'

Luise's story is a personal portrayal, but I have chosen to cast it in a wider context.

Writing this book has been a somber task, as I cannot fully express my feelings of impotence and grief. Words turn to stone when I try to describe what she and others like her have been subjected to. You have to feel it in your own body.

But Luise's story is significant, even though it is heartbreaking. If I don't tell the story, it would be as though it never happened.

It did happen, and these untimely, unnatural deaths will continue as long as politicians and ordinary people turn a blind eye.

I hope this book promotes reflection on this human rights issue.

A big thank you to all who have supported me with advice and encouragement through this difficult process.

Apart from friends and acquaintances, the characters in this book have been given different names.

Dorrit Cato Christensen

1

July 15, 2005

I love the sunlit early summer mornings.

I am in that meditative state halfway between REM sleep and wakefulness.

A sunbeam has crept in through a gap in the blue curtains and landed on my left cheek.

It warms my soul.

The hoarse cry of the magpies outside my window tells me they are happily engaged in their favorite pastime, teasing the downstairs neighbor's stoical cat, Hannibal. Their ingenious maneuvers goad the unfortunate creature to scamper back and forth, as if in a cage.

The birds strut quietly in front of the Hannibal, tails bobbing. Hannibal runs at them but at the last moment they take flight and immediately land on his other side, squawking. Hannibal looks around bewildered and catches sight of the magpies behind him. They totter quietly away, the cat runs after them, and the frolic is repeated until Hannibal gives up, humiliated.

In my meditative state I have an imaginary talk with Luise about the magpie incident. She's very familiar with the routine. We've always been amazed how Hannibal gets sucked into their game every time. As Luise would say, 'Hannibal is doing his morning exercise again. He's probably addicted.'

I lie there, waiting for 1:00 pm, when I will be visiting Luise in the psychiatric ward at Amager Hospital. Even the locked doors and body searches cannot diminish my joy at seeing her.

Two weeks before, Luise had been transferred to a secure intensive care ward. The psychiatrists now think Luise poses a danger to others.

I know there's nothing to this.

Being stuck in this chaotic ward terrifies Luise, but that problem is solved with a whole lot of extra drugs to deal with the anxiety.

The phone rings at 6:30 am and tears me out of my dreamlike state.

I just begin to think: 'Luise doesn't usually call this early.'

It's not Luise. It's a doctor from Amager Hospital calling to tell me Luise is dead.

I hear myself scream.

2

APRIL 29, 2002

This was the day I started to write what would become this book. Why exactly this day? Luise's consultation with her psychiatrist had more or less the same result as always.

I can see from your journal how you have insisted over the years that you cannot tolerate the medication and have requested a lower dose. The psychiatrist always answered that you were very ill and would get even worse if you didn't go along with his treatment. It's clear you were never taken seriously, and since you didn't want to defy authority you always complied. Nothing new there.

I have said over the years that the strong doses of medication were making you ill. You got anxiety attacks, had hallucinations, and became distraught. The higher the dose, the worse your torment. I often said that if the dose wasn't reduced, things would end badly. I've also learned that my 'intervention' in your treatment in several cases led to even higher doses. Anyway, the consultation with your psychiatrist on April 29 2002 was just like most previous sessions. But this was the first time I saw you after the consult. It struck me hard to see how badly it had affected you.

We were at Sundbygård, Luise's residential treatment home. We sat in the hallway waiting for her to talk to Sofus, her psychiatrist. Afterwards we were going to Holbæk to celebrate grandma's 89th birthday.

We sat and chatted. Luise said: 'I'm looking forward to our coffee break in Roskilde.' Then her gurgling laughter. The coffee break in Roskilde was our standing joke about DSB, the Danish rail system. DSB operation was often erratic, so we sometimes had to change in Roskilde to a Holbæk train. We would have coffee in Roskilde while waiting for a connection. When the train went according to plan, directly to Holbæk, Luise often said with a wry smile: 'Arrgh! There goes our coffee break.'

Normally she wanted me to talk to her psychiatrist on her behalf. She knew from bitter experience that she always lost the argument. The psychiatrist did not listen to what she said, and he did not accept her request for a lower dose of the medication.

Today, for once, she dared to have the consultation with Sofus by herself, because the outcome was inevitable. She should be given a lower dose of the antipsychotic drug Orap (Pimozid). She believed the conversation was just a formality.

After three weeks at Amager Hospital Luise was discharged on April 10, 2002. During the hospitalization it was decided that she would slowly be taken off Orap.

Extract from the April 8 chart note from Amager Hospital:
'The patient is advised that dosage reduction will take place at Sundbygård. For a start I am complying with her wish to lower Orap dosage, and she is reduced to 12 mg.'

Your contact person from your residential care home and your psychiatrist had both participated in the conference at Amager Hospital on April 9, when a further decrease in the Orap dose was confirmed.

So everybody knew that treatment with this drug was being phased out.

We sat and waited outside the meeting room. Luise sparkled. She was wearing her beautiful eggplant-colored silk pants and a loose silk blouse that matched the pants. It was Luise's favorite outfit, which she had bought the year before in Portland, Oregon. The clothes brought out the colors of her beaming face.

In her hands she had a bouquet of red roses. 'Grandmother must have red roses because I love her.'

You were looking forward to a psychiatric consultation where your request for less medication would for once be honored. A conversation where you would be heard and taken seriously.

You walked into the room with head held high and came out shortly afterwards stiff and gray.

Excerpts of chart notes for the April 29 consult:
'Conversation with patient. She expresses a desire to reduce the Orap dose ... In the session I recommend she should continue with Orap unchanged, which she seems to accept ...'

Your expression and slumping posture as you came out of the consultation did not indicate that you had voluntarily accepted.

You told me, 'Sofus will not let me reduce the Orap. You must go and talk to him, Mom.'

I went in and asked Sofus why he would not reduce Luise's Orap dosage, as had been decided a few weeks earlier while she was being treated at Amager Hospital. The result of my efforts was that instead of coming off the medication, her dosage was to be increased.

I was cold and stiff as I walked out of the consulting room. My legs barely functioned – I could hardly put one foot in front of the other. I walked with head erect, my forehead so upright that my whole body was bent backwards. This was the only way I could get my reluctant limbs to work.

I felt the urge to scream and lash out wildly around me. But a calm mother doesn't do that kind of thing.

Waiting outside the consulting room, you looked expectantly at me.

'What did Sofus say?' you asked.

My small voice uttered soothing words: 'Sofus thinks it's best for you if you take more medicine.'

You got angry and shouted: 'Get out of here. I don't want to see you anymore. You're not helping me. You've never helped me. You always say the same as them. They're killing me with their drugs, and you just don't care. Get out!'

Your anger was understandably directed against me. The red roses for grandmother were thrown on the floor.

You did not come to grandma's 89th birthday.

Instead, you spent the rest of the day in bed under heavy sedation.

I didn't get to grandma's birthday either. I tried to make myself go, but I was heartbroken.

It was neither the first nor the last time we would be in a situation where you had blind faith in my ability to help you, only to see your situation take a turn for the worse.

I was crushed. I could not bear the thought that I had again disappointed Luise.

I came home crying. I wrote and wrote. My desperation made the words incoherent. The expression on Luise's face when she came out of the consult with Sofus was etched in my mind. It took over my entire body like a big painful boil. To think that in a five-minute consultation a psychiatrist could transform a bright, erect woman into a pale-gray girl with dead eyes and that characteristic drug-induced stoop.

I had done everything in my power. At the same time I got a nasty feeling that Sofus' 'show of force' with the increased medication dose had nothing to do with Luise's welfare, but rather was intended to demonstrate who was making the decisions. Sad to relate, this was not the first time I experienced such a power play in the psychiatric treatment system.

Over the years I contacted I don't know how many experts in hopes of meeting someone who could come up with the right kind of support for

Luise. I tried to get help through Social Services. For several years I tried the dialog approach – family consultations with the treating psychiatrists. Since the talks changed nothing – and even made things worse – I started to write letters to air my concerns over Luise's medical treatment, which I thought was reckless and consistently made her worse.

I began to see a psychiatrist myself, wondering whether it was perhaps my fault that everything went wrong, that it was my personal input that caused my relationship with psychiatrists to fall apart, so that Luise's treatment never got on the right track. I hoped that the therapy sessions might get me better prepared, so I could communicate with Luise's psychiatrists.

Nothing helped.

As time passed I was consumed by sorrow. I felt inept and paralyzed.

It pained me endlessly to feel like a passive spectator watching Luise's mistreatment in a mental health system that was unaccountable, rigid and aloof.

But it pained me even more that Luise thought I didn't want to help her.

April 29, 2002: Dear Luise, I understand that you felt I did not help you today with Sofus.

I want you to see that I tried.

I can see why you often get angry at me and accuse me of never wanting to help you. But I can't understand why so soon after your accusations you apologize. Your anger is justified. I have not always helped you well enough.

But, dear Luise, it's important that you realize I'm doing my best, that through the years I've desperately tried everything in my power to help you.

Unfortunately, everything in my power is not always enough.

And I'm very sorry about that.

But you don't need a mother who's sad, you need a mother you can have good and happy experiences with. And we've had many wonderful experiences together.

Do you remember our trips to New Zealand, USA, Palestine, Spain, Greece and especially our annual trips to London and Cornwall? Haven't we been to many wonderful places and met many nice people?

Yes, we have done many things together, enjoyed ourselves and laughed. We have a special connection, you and I – all we have to do is just look at each other to know what the other person is thinking or laughing about.

Luise, I want to tell you about all your incredible abilities – because everything you can't do has been firmly nailed down with six-inch nails.

You have marvelous inner strength. You don't give up. You have a great appetite for life and a desire to experience the world. I think your humor, your strength and your thirst for experience make your life a good one. In spite of everything.

I don't understand where you get your strength from, and I am full of admiration for your enthusiasm. You know how hard it is to be constantly misunderstood. You have experienced first hand how bad things can get when you don't fit into society's little boxes. You've often said you wanted to tell about your experiences in the hope that it would help other people.

3

I AM NOT MENTALLY ILL

*They are a colorful thread in life's precious patchwork.
Our civilization would be extremely dull and sterile
if we didn't have people with Asperger's syndrome
and didn't know how to appreciate them.*

Tony Attwood

'I am not mentally ill – I have Asperger's' was the headline to an article in the in the September/October 2004 issue of the Danish psychiatry magazine Outsideren, *You asked me to read the article, saying, 'Mom, this could be me!'*

The article tells about a young man diagnosed with schizophrenia who over a ten-year period had multiple admissions to psychiatric units, where he was treated with large doses of antipsychotic medication. After ten years in a drug hell, he was fortunate enough to come across a psychiatrist who could see that the schizophrenia diagnosis was wrong and that he actually suffered from Asperger's syndrome.

The antipsychotic medication was discontinued. He finishes the article: 'I've been told that on top of the Asperger's I suffer from a mild form of schizophrenia. But the psychiatrist who tested me thought it was the result of years of medication with antipsychotic drugs.'

You're right, it could have been you.

You were not schizophrenic either. But all those psychiatrists wouldn't recognize this. Why on earth couldn't they see this?

When it comes to health care, we all get the same random draw. Some of us get lucky and find a competent, sympathetic practitioner who listens carefully so he/she can arrive at the right treatment.

Luise, you weren't so lucky.

Your pained cry to me on April 29, 2002, was woefully right: 'They're killing me with their drugs.'

August 29, 1972.

Luise. I want you to know that you were born in love.

On August 29 is a special day in Danish history, as several well-wishers reminded us. On this day in 1943 the wartime Danish government ended its cooperation with the German occupiers.

For us it was the day you came into the world. Our joy made everything else pale into insignificance.

You were really wanted.

Your father and I had already chosen your name.

You would be named Suzanne or Nikoline.

But when you showed yourself to the world, you were a ready-made Luise.

It's strange that, at first sight of a half-hour old baby girl, we could say, 'She's a Luise.' But it was true, and Luise became your name.

Martin and I wanted you to have the most heavenly and natural childhood. We were young people of the Sixties. Our educational role model was based on the child-rearing practices of primitive peoples. This meant from the start that you were destined to be a fully paid-up member of our world. You were going to live with us and experience life with us.

We would wait as long as possible before we let you go to kindergarten, so you could develop at your own pace, living full-time with us.

We believed the old ideas about serenity, structure and cleanliness should be downgraded in favor of the principle that you needed to share everything with us – and, we fondly imagined, exactly on our own terms.

We were certain that children are always better off of living with their parents, for good or ill – a belief based on love.

Ideological principles are one thing. Living them is quite another. It seems we somehow forgot, without even noticing it, that you were supposed to share our daily rhythm.

Anyway, Martin and I suddenly found it entirely normal to be sitting drinking tea between 2 am and 4 am. We did this because you usually woke up around that time and obviously liked to be entertained.

But otherwise.

If we were visiting friends or family for the evening, you had to either stay up until we got home or fall asleep at our host's. We believed our child-rearing style would turn you into a healthy, creative and reflective girl.

We all hit the road and travelled to Morocco when you were three months old. Lived in small hotels and had a wonderful time for two months. It was one of those times all three of us loved being together. You were the center of attention without ever asking to be. Although we assumed you were just tagging along on our trip, it was in fact we who were following you.

We spent the days walking and relaxing. Sitting under the palm trees, eating bread and drinking juice.

You were only little then. Even with your photographic memory you probably don't remember, but you knew you were part of that togetherness.

You probably don't even remember me rocking you and singing:

You are my sunshine, my only sunshine

You make me happy, when skies are grey

You'll never know dear, how much I love you

Please don't take my sunshine away.

You were moving your head to the beat of my song, so I know you got it.

Luise, you had a powerful voice. If you cried because you were hungry or wet, we had to deal with it immediately.

Your father had a hard time coping and found it almost impossible to comfort you as you shrieked at full pitch.

You have always been a wonderful girl, but full of contrasts. On the one hand, you seemed happy and confident, eager to explore all of life's mysteries, and you were braver than most. On the other hand, inside you lurked that easily aroused anxiety, which was evident from the day you were born.

You were very sensitive to sounds. The noise from car horns, road drills and vacuum cleaners would upset you and bring out your heart-rending cry.

At the hospital the nurses were tough. In the early 1970s it was unimaginable for a mother to bring her newborn baby into bed with her.

You would have loved that, and so would I.

But no. You could only lie with me when you were nursing. Then it was back to your cold little cot. The rule was not up for discussion.

Those tough nurses used to say: 'Babies are best off lying in their own little bed.' Maybe the practice was best for babies in the early 1970s. But it certainly isn't today.

Thinking has also changed with regard to children's sleep routine.

You never wanted to be alone in your bed. It was uncomfortable and cold.

Sometimes your loud crying would peel through the ward.

I was carefully instructed to be resolute and leave you to cry yourself to sleep. That way you could learn how to lie there alone, according to the nurses.

I didn't like the idea at all, nor did you, as you didn't fall asleep anyway.

September 2, 1972, we finally brought you home.

It was just past noon when we walked across Fælledparken's big green meadow with our blue baby carriage, which was beautifully painted with many-colored flowers.

We were on our way home to Brumleby. Your father and I were proud and happy beyond measure – there you were in the baby carriage, our priceless jewel. The sun shone from a cloudless sky – at least I think it did. The sun was shining in my head anyway. Martin's freshly painted flowers on our used pram were a delight to the eye. I felt sure our happiness lit up the park. There were no dark clouds that day.

It was good to come home, where no one else could decide who should lie in which bed.

Our dear cat Tulipip, however, was not excited at your homecoming. He quickly realized he would now be number two in the hierarchy. With a derisive flip of the tail he walked out on us, never to return. He moved in with the next-door neighbors.

Whenever you wanted to be held, I soon learned it was best just to pick you up immediately. Otherwise you would complain until I ended up doing it anyway. I had bought a baby snuggler so you could be next to my chest. It was wonderful to walk around with you next to me while doing the daily chores.

Sometimes you cried a lot. The nurse called it colic, but colic doesn't last for eighteen months.

All the good nurses and honorary aunts told me it was just a question of being steadfast and letting you scream when put to bed. Eventually you would cry yourself to sleep. I was just being too soft, they said.

All their well-meaning advice didn't help. One time we tried to let you cry for what seemed like hours. When we finally gave up, you were inconsolable for the rest of the evening.

Then I realized public health nurses and aunts are not always right.

I'm perhaps making it sound like you were always crying, but that's certainly not the case.

You also had long periods where you could happily spend hours sitting and babbling, playing by yourself or with me.

But when you cried, it was as if your tears were caused by an inexplicable sense of insecurity that suddenly overpowered you. I could feel your pain, but I couldn't figure out what was tormenting you so terribly on these occasions.

But most of the time you were a charming and happy little girl.

You could entertain a whole crowd. You could give people looks that would crack them up. By the time you were one you had started to have fun mimicking people's facial expressions. I'll never forget the time we sat at our neighbor Trine's, knitting and chattering. Inge, another neighbor, was there too. The three of us often got together, and you loved Trine and Inge. Suddenly, in a loud voice you began to mimic us. You grabbed my knitting, sat down and rocked back and forth, knitting needles clattering, while talking gibberish and laughing.

You knew how to modulate your voice to impersonate each one of us.

This love of impersonating people carried over into your adult life.

Some of Luise's favorite TV comedy shows were *Linie 3* (Line 3) and *De Nattergale* (which in Danish can mean The Nightingales or The Crazy Night People). She used *Linie 3*'s satire of the well-known Danish politician Erhard Jakobsen, former Mayor of Gladsaxe, on several occasions.

Luise could sound like Jakobsen when she burst out: 'I never said that. What did you never say? What I just said.'

Not to mention the party we threw many years ago, where the discussion got rather unpleasantly intense.

Luise redeemed the situation with one of Preben Kristensen's stunts from *Linie 3.*

She swept majestically into the kitchen where we sat, wearing old-fashioned clothes and a big hat.

She had a rose in her hand. Mimicking Queen Margrethe's voice (the Queen of Denmark is a fully qualified archeologist), she delivered the pun-laden Danish equivalent of: 'I've just been to Egypt. Oh, it was just the pits – the sand pits.'

Her entrance was timed perfectly and the tense mood lifted.

Luise, by the time you were two and three years old you were quite comfortable with people you didn't know.

I watched your peers being a little nervous and hesitant in their dealings with strangers. But you walked straight into people's hearts. Our friends stood in line to look after you.

Your spirit of adventure was evident from when you began to walk. Often it took the form of explorations that took you too far and wide for your age. You loved to wander by yourself and discover things. You were never fretful when you 'got lost.'

Can you remember when we were in Crete with Bjarne and

Trine, our wonderful neighbors from Brumleby? You were three.

We stayed in a small mountain village, where we rented a house – without beds or furniture, as it turned out.

You went off visiting people in the village. Our new neighbors started to drop by to check in on you and bring you cookies. They saw there was no furniture in the house. Then each of them returned with bits of furniture so our house became almost habitable.

Then one morning you vanished.

The four of us searched in every direction, climbing up and down among the rocks. We combed the area without success. We were all aware of the one place we had been avoiding.

It was a very steep slope that dropped several meters.

But it was the last possible place to look.

We were all worried we might make a horrible discovery.

But that didn't happen – quite the contrary.

There you stood at the bottom of the rock face with a big smile: 'Hi! It's hard to get up out of here.'

The front of your blouse was stained red brown from the Cretan soil, a clear sign that you, Sisyphus-like, had tried to clamber up the cliff several times and slipped back down.

You saw this predicament as an exciting challenge.

After Bjarne and Trine left, we met Nick, Jane and little Jes from New Zealand. You and Jes were the same age and played well together. Your father and I both had the thought that here was a good chance for you to learn English at an early age.

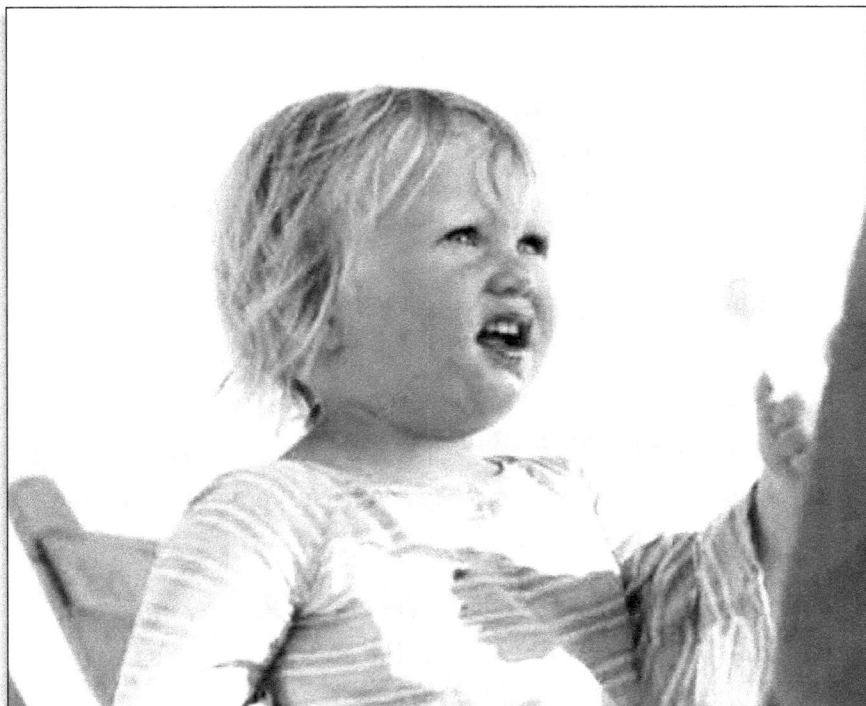

Luise in Majorca at age two

But you had other plans.

You made sure you and Jes could communicate in Danish.

You didn't learn English until later. On the other hand, Jes was well equipped language-wise when the family later came to Denmark and stayed with us for three months.

When you were five years old your father left and the two of us started travelling alone.

We traveled to England and other places every summer to visit friends.

I recall with horror our first trip alone when you managed to slip out of my hand at Oxford Circus in London.

You had disappeared. And there were a hell of a lot of places to search at this busy intersection.

There must have been ten people helping me look for you.

We found you after what seemed like hours.

Finally you appeared, cheerfully walking along holding a lady's hand not far from Oxford Circus. The lady was looking for a policeman, because she couldn't take you home with her.

I ran up and asked melodramatically: 'Weren't you afraid?'

'Why?' you asked. 'I was just taking a walk with the lady.'

A stupid question on my part. You looked quite content. I was the one that was scared.

On the one hand, I was glad you felt comfortable with strangers. But at the same time I was nervous about where your unconditional trust might lead.

The long lone wanderings, where you ended up lost, also worried me. It was clear your little friends didn't need to experience life like you. They might roam far and wide but always made sure their parents were never out of sight – and if they lost sight of them they usually got scared and started to cry.

You had no such limitations.

Your fearlessness stood in stark contrast to the inner anxiety that troubled you at times. Some nights you were kept up by night-mares and could only fall asleep in my bed.

4

CHILDHOOD IN BRUMLEBY

Our little-bitty houses might be short on space.
But right outside there's always room for every face.
You don't see many cars in Brumleby, you know.
No one gets run over, so our numbers grow and grow.
Refrain:
There's lots of kids in Brumleby and we're all treated well.
If someone tries to kick us out, we'll kick 'em all to hell.

Free translation of the 'Children's Song'
for the 1978 Brumleby Cabaret

Can you remember when you performed the children's song at our annual cabaret in 1978?

You did a beautiful job. Later that year we were at the Metronome sound studio to record the song. You guys were so good. The song went public on the Brumleby album the following year.

The Brumleby neighborhood was like a village where everyone knew each other and the doors were always open. With no through streets and few vehicles, it was (and remains) a very safe environment for both children and adults.

We staged a performance twice a year, the cabaret every autumn and the children's theater at our spring festival. For the 1977 spring bash we produced a very successful clown sketch. You and Rasmus were clowns, and Anni and I were clown mothers and coaches. The number was backed by our local 'Brumleorchestra.' You two five-year-old clowns cavorted on stage, sang songs, bumped into each other and rolled around in a very disciplined way.

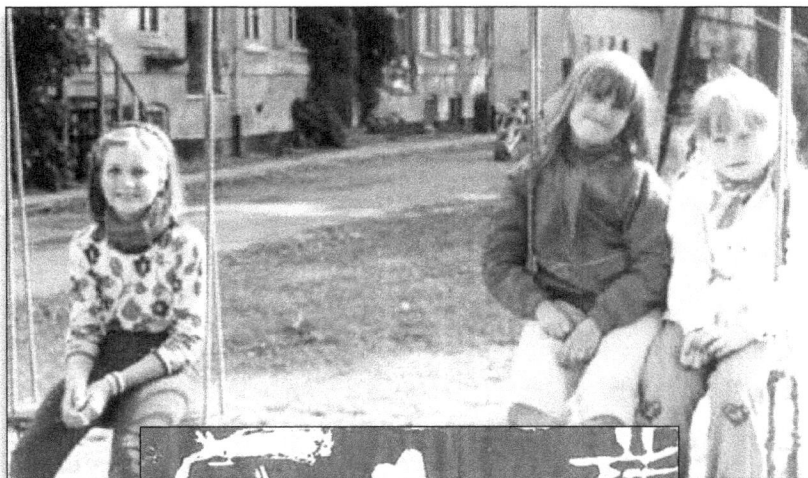

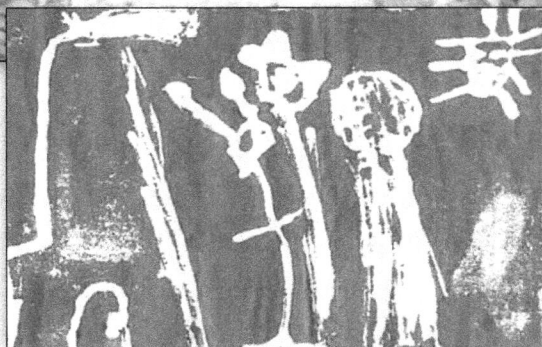

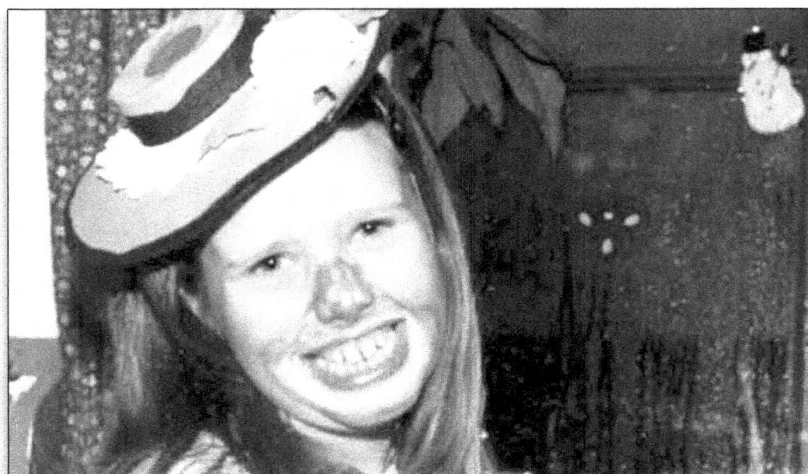

Luise with friends Kia and Laila in Brumleby; one of her linoleum cuts from age seven; all dressed up for a theatrical skit.

The performance's climax came when you had to sit at a table and eat a whole layer cake, covered in whipped cream, of course. Anni and I were responsible for an unfortunate technical error. The chairs you were to sit in had no seat bottom. The audience couldn't see this as there was a rug over the seats.

At rehearsals the chairs did have proper seats, so we didn't expect you to get totally stuck when you sat in the seat holes during the live performance.

But you handled the situation with great resourcefulness, crawling around on all fours, chairs stuck on your butts, uttering clownish complaints. It all looked very special, with the upturned chair legs waving in the air.

The sketch turned out much funnier than planned.

Do you remember the time we made the 60 layer cakes? This was during the 1983 spring festival. The weather was glorious and we got far more visitors than expected. We had to call in reinforcements to help with cake production.

By the time we closed our layer cake stall at 5 pm we were falling about laughing. This was partly due to fatigue, but also because we were more or less covered in whipped cream, cake icing and jam.

From the time you were very small you brought playmates to our house. You all loved staging plays, and you in particular were very good at initiating these theatrical productions.

Some of your friends were very inventive, and the gang could turn the house upside down in no time flat.

When you and Tobias would play together and suddenly start laughing in a particular way, I knew trouble was brewing. One time I walked into the kitchen to find you'd emptied bags of flour and sugar all over the floor and then topped it with pickled beets!

You two thought this was hilarious. Me not so much.

Tobias was not scared to light matches, and you admired him for this. Then one day I heard ominous laughter coming from the living room. I arrived to find a toilet paper bonfire blazing away.

This minor case of arson was not serious. You were five years old, and the flames had not spread. The funny thing was that Tobias said it was you who had lit the fire. You didn't deny it. Tobias was standing there holding the matchbox, so you perhaps didn't think further debate was needed to determine who the culprit was.

Such little white lies were not your style, however. You more often ended up with hurt feelings.

Whenever kids did something 'bad' in Brumleby, your playmates would immediately deny any responsibility. When asked if you were the culprit, you would respond evasively. So you got scolded.

I never understood why you reacted this way, but I had a feeling that you could not figure out how to stand up for yourself.

Another explanation may be that you were so hurt at being subject to an obviously unfair accusation that you saw no point in defending yourself.

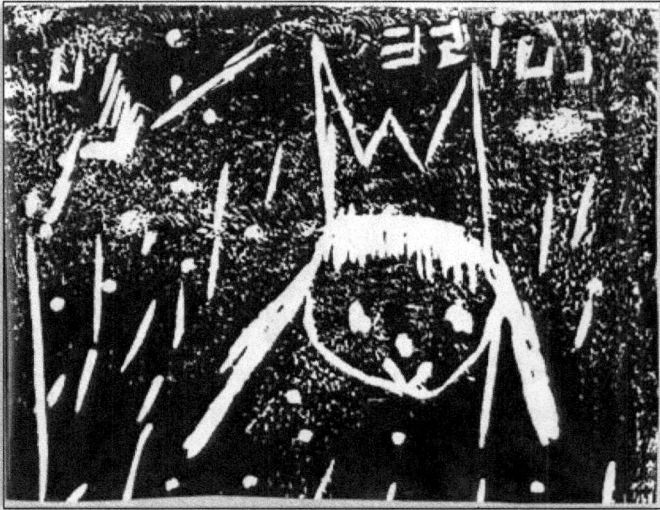

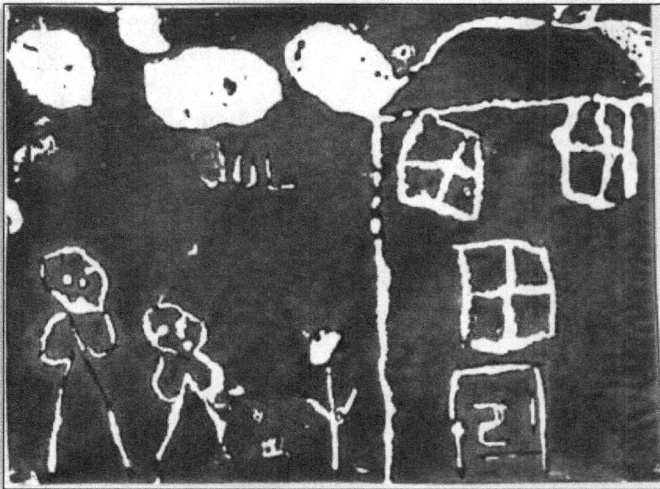

Mom's favorite linoleum cut and a Christmas painting.

5

KINDERGARTEN

Little cat, little cat,
Walking so alone.
Tell me whose cat you are?
I'm damn well my own.

Piet Hein

Your father and I had always planned to wait as long as possible before sending you to pre-school. We realized you were not the kind of group-oriented kid who could easily fit in at kindergarten. You preferred unstructured play. You were your own person, and you were wonderful at it.

But unfortunately we had to make money, something your father was not always good at. Though he was very smart, his work life was never particularly stable.

In your first year I did odd jobs where you could stay with me, and I also did childcare for others. When you were two and a half we had to bite the bullet and send you to kindergarten. I got a job with fixed working hours.

As a qualified teacher, I was all too familiar with the educational ideologies of the 1970s, which were partially inspired by the idea of the 'self-governing child collective,' as advocated by the then-famous Soviet pedagogue Anton Semenovych Makarenko.

Group-oriented education was the favored norm, stressing personal responsibility and accountability.

In Denmark in the 1970s, this educational philosophy of group-oriented child-rearing had a major influence on children's social activities and day care experiences. The very nature of collective effort was seen as an important educational tool.

Every day, Luise, you had to sit through the morning meeting with a large bunch of kids with whom you were supposed to socialize and collaboratively plan the day's activities. Good heavens, you weren't yet three and you simply couldn't see the purpose of this half-hour get-together. The teacher held you in his power, he was hell-bent on ensuring that you all worked happily together and decided things like who should be awarded 'adult tasks' such as washing the group's ten cups in the tiny sink.

Your dishwashing day was Tuesday. Every Tuesday you faithfully carried the cups out to the dishwasher in the kitchen. Your logic told you this was a sensible solution to the task at hand. But no way! You had to stand on the plinth and wash up those ten cups by hand every Tuesday, because this had been decided at the morning meeting in the holy name of collective education and collective decision-making.

You loved to do the dishes, but not just on Tuesdays. You would have loved to wash cups on Wednesdays or Thursdays, but you weren't allowed to.

The staff insisted you comply. But you didn't conform, and cried when subjected to this show of force.

The teachers' initiative to keep you stuck in the cozy breakfast meetings, with a dishwashing day on Tuesday, caused you great pain. You seemed to experience it almost like a violation.

The kindergarten referred us to a family counselor. You were four at the time.

We were discharged after the second session. But the psychologist dropped by your daycare one day – she wanted to get an idea of what your everyday life was like.

The psychologist later told me the kindergarten had written in their referral note to her: 'The mother has indicated she cannot handle having her daughter at home.' The psychologist could clearly see this was not true. She suggested it would be best for you to switch to a new daycare center. Her reason was that these educational practices were not suitable for you.

So you started at the new nursery school, where the teaching was less 'militaristic' and you quickly grew to like the new conditions.

Here you were allowed to help in the kitchen as much as you liked, washing dishes and doing useful tasks.

You were always a helpful girl. You loved to lend a hand with cleaning, setting the table, cooking and general housework. Mostly anyway, because sometimes you could go into a sudden mental lockdown and refuse to help. If we kept pushing, you got mad.

I might ask: 'Would you bring me the milk from the fridge?' If you answered no, it didn't help if I tried persuading you with 'Please get the milk for me.' It helped even less if I tried to get tough on you. Because you weren't going to fetch the milk once you had said no. Further discussion was useless.

6

SCENE CHANGE

*You could still understand
even when things turned weird,
and you got angry with yourself,
or got angry with me
because I spoke too harshly to you.*

I had learned by now that if you said no, I should refrain from repeating my request and just wait. Then you would do the job anyway.

For you, the road to this realization was littered with conflict and defeat.

I tried over a long period to be persistent in my requests to you, to show I was the one who made the decisions. I never managed to get this through to you. The more I put my foot down, the more you defied me. This didn't result in your becoming more docile – in fact, it made you unhappy. I could see in your eyes that you didn't say no just to test limits, that you actually didn't understand why I scolded you, and that you ultimately interpreted all this as my not loving you.

After much floundering I found a way to get around the 'saying no' problem. I learned that whenever I appealed to your sense of humor your negativity would disappear. When I talked to you in a light-hearted, non-accusatory tone, you were totally at ease.

I called it our scene change. We could, for example, sit down for breakfast with no milk on the table. I would start to fantasize about whether the milk for our cornflakes might magically make *its way over to the table. We could sit and laugh, and then you would go and fetch the stubborn milk. Our joking around with each other lifted the mood, and you handled the task.*

Our daily conflicts diminished after I implemented my scene change approach, which enabled us to solve many problems with humor.

But this didn't help you in an institutional environment where staff followed meticulous guidelines on how children should develop at different ages. If children didn't meet the requirements appropriate to their age, powerful means could be deployed to make sure they did.

As a trained teacher, I could see that the methods that worked so positively for many children had an adverse effect on sensitive children like you.

You were already quite attuned to adult body language, which sometimes signaled to you that grown-ups were irritated by your stubbornness. Their consequent assumption that you were going to defy them often meant that they then addressed you in a more forceful, frosty tone.

Your teachers' tone of voice became a contributory factor to your tendency to clam up and say no. You became unhappy and often asked me: 'Why doesn't anyone like me at kindergarten? The grown-ups always get mad at me.'

Luise, far too much emphasis was put on the things your teachers thought you should be able to do – but which you simply couldn't do. By contrast, it was rare that staff realized that you could actually do many things beyond your age level. But they did use you as a helper on school field trips. They would say: 'Luise is very good at keeping the wild children in line. She acts confident in busy road conditions, and this rubs off on the more unruly children.'

I once read an amusing article in the daily newspaper *Politiken* dealing with this obsession with the minutiae of a child's development. The piece was headlined 'Olga's state-controlled learning process':

'Congratulations! It's a girl. Here's the punch card that will forever follow your little Olga on her long journey through the state's new educational system towards the common goal. Olga's parents celebrate. What do we know about children's lives today? A good thing the state knows better. So Olga's learning process gets off to a great start. On the health nurse's first visit it's determined that Olga can successfully burp, in accordance with the nationally developed baby test. Actually, having burped twice, Olga is overqualified for a place at the crèche. This is entered in Olga's personal test results and pointed out to the nursery staff by two justly proud parents. At 10:45 am in March Olga also passed the 'standing on tip-toe' test. She passed every test in the nursery with flying colors. But problems became apparent in kindergarten. Here the nationally imposed learning milestones were difficult for Olga to reach. These included learning how stick a fork in a difficult potato, which she finally accomplished. But she also had to learn how to tie her own shoes. This was almost a disaster, but thankfully Olga was granted an exemption because she was not yet five when she started the test. Her parents breathed a sigh of relief. Olga was allowed to enter pre-school. But the punch card detailed her problem with shoelaces in nursery school. Olga would have to undergo daily shoelace training in private before she could become a full-fledged member of the community. Then they would let her join the other children and learn to sit quietly and listen to small bits of information. Numbers and letters bounced off little Olga, who would rather be playing Mommy and Daddy with little freckle-faced Ivan.'

I got tired of hearing from teachers and family friends that I was being too permissive. 'If you do such and such, then Luise will do as she's told.' I know the advice was well-meant, but I had already tried it. Experience had taught me that our 'scene change' procedure worked best.

This doesn't mean I was never receptive to parenting tips. I certainly was, since I knew I hadn't found the Philosopher's Stone.

Lars, a family friend for many years, was sure that it was simply a matter of defeating your 'no monster.' He said: 'We shouldn't be permissive. It makes children uncertain.' His two boys were fully functioning and nice to be around.

I let Lars try to leap in, starting with the familiar 'please get the milk' scenario. He first tried persuasion and predictably failed. Then he gave her a smack on the butt, and sternly insisted she comply. But she was unmoved: 'No way!'

I must admit that it startled me when he spanked her. I had never even laid a hand on Luise. But I thought, 'Maybe a tap on the butt might work wonders.'

Lars quickly regretted his attempt at strict child-rearing, which in any case didn't produce a positive outcome. He tried to make things right by offering you a 10-kroner coin (about $2). You threw it back in his face. Then he offered to buy you an ice cream, which you refused. You'd lost trust in Lars.

Luise, you always remembered people who were good to you – and you certainly remembered people who had treated you badly.

The next time Lars came to see us you were sitting on the doorstep eating peas. Lars asked for a pea. You simply said no. He offered to buy one, but you were unmoved. You stood up to confront him, hands on hips and head tilted, and said: 'Tell me, have you already forgotten that you actually hit me?' You said it almost exultantly, with a wry smile and a twinkle in your eye.

Lars apologized.

He got the pea.

You got your redress for the humiliation he had visited on you – with the best intentions, of course – because you wouldn't get milk from the fridge. You wouldn't accept money as payment for the demeaning treatment. You wanted an apology.

You got your apology and accepted it. You bore no grudge. Your response in many ways was totally adult.

7

STARTING SCHOOL

*The day finally arrived in 1979
for you to start school.
Your big pink school backpack
had stood at your bedside for two months.
It had been re-packed almost daily.
You were proud, excited and eager.*

Luise had been looking forward to this for the past six months. The pink satchel from grandpa had been packed and ready for two months. It contained a very sophisticated pencil case that had three levels and countless little compartments that sprang open at the press of a button. There were slots for five erasers, pencil sharpeners, a myriad of color-fully decorated pencils, and whatever else was in vogue. She could have packed most of her room in that school bag.

Luise got up early. She had to repack the bag just one more time. Maybe she shouldn't bring Teddy along to school, but perhaps her doll Tina could come?

The sun shone from a cloudless sky as we walked down Randers Street to the school.

Four of her friends from Brumleby were starting in the same class. They had all compared school bags and traded pencils and erasers while waiting for the big day. School was always in the air.

We parents at first took turns walking them all to school. But it was not long before they could get there by themselves.

At first they all sat as quiet as mice, ready to soak up knowledge. After the novelty wore off and they realized they couldn't start reading comics, things started to turn more rowdy in the classroom.

Luise was smart but easily bothered by the noise and commotion, so much so that she had trouble concentrating amid the growing boisterousness, which in turn meant that the pace of her learning fluctuated.

Things quickly started going downhill, especially in math. The math teacher's teaching style was not geared to her. He made her anxious. At first-grade parents' day I sat in on the math class. It was a disheartening experience. She was called to the blackboard with the words: 'Now we'll see if Luise can handle this difficult task.' She was supposed to add two plus two. But the teacher's momentary eye-rolling and ironic tone of voice signaled the expectation that she absolutely could not handle it. It was humiliating and degrading. She was nervous and, as usual, froze. The whole class found it funny.

I asked for a meeting with the school principal to discuss the math teacher's teaching method, or rather lack thereof. At the meeting I didn't even get to make my point before he threw in my face: 'What are you doing wrong, are you too strict with Luise or are you spoiling her too much?' I was very surprised and disconcerted, and could only answer: 'I don't know'. His question made it clear that the school did not take my concerns seriously.

We left the house at the same time every morning, she going to school and me heading for work. Sometimes this could cause problems. She had a growing distaste for school, particularly math.

Mostly, though, we got out of the house without a problem.

A few years back I put a tape in the machine that had Bob Marley's 'Babylon' on it, one of my favorite tracks.

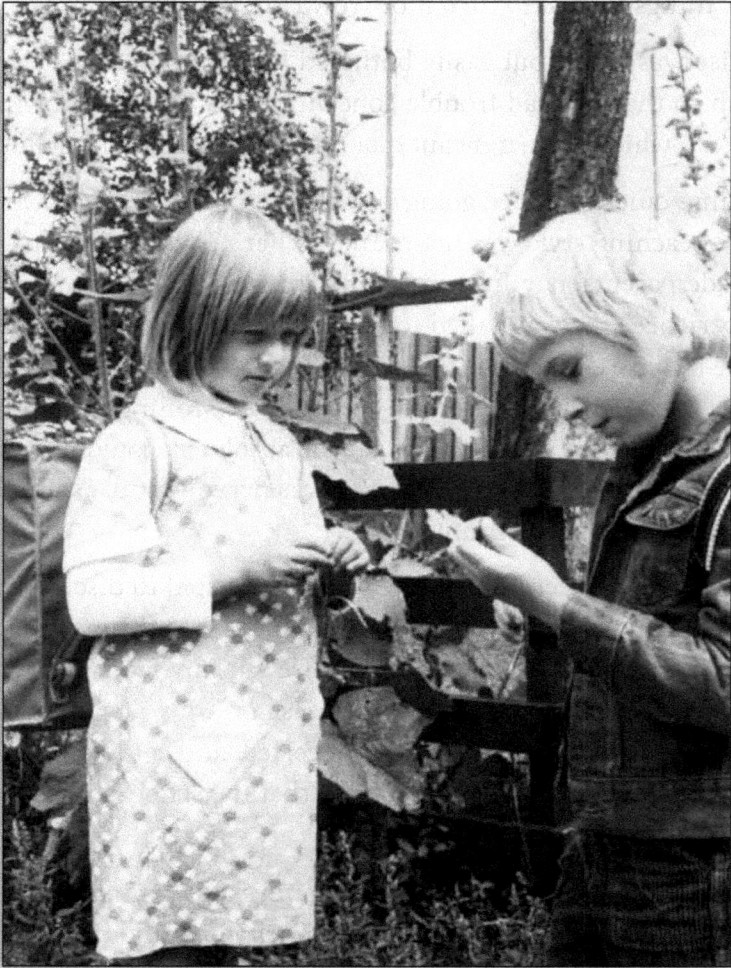

Luise, with backpack, off to the first day of school with Jonas.

But it wasn't Bob Marley's reggae that came out of the speakers – a Luise and Dorrit morning session was recorded over it. The theme was her refusal to go to school:

'Luise we have to go now.'

'No, I'm not going to school today.'

'Well, you have to, because I have to go to work.'

'I'm not going to school, I don't want math with that stupid math teacher. He's always on my case.'

I shout a long: 'Lui-i-i-ise. We'd better go now.' To my surprise, my voice doesn't sound the slightest bit irritated.

Abrupt scene change as you shout: 'Mommm!'

'Yes, what is it?'

She answers with a clever children's pun, untranslatable from the Danish, and then her gurgling laughter.

Again, she was now the one to change the scene and elevate the mood.

So off we went to school and work.

She loved to record conversations without our knowing it. She made some brilliant collages of sound bites from different conversations interspersed with music.

How I miss you. How I miss your delightfully infectious laughter.

8

AFTERSCHOOL CENTER

The little prince said of his rose:
'She means more to me than all of you...
Because it is she that I have watered...
Because it is she I have listened to...
Even sometimes when she said nothing.
Because she is my rose.'

Antoine de Saint-Exupéry *The Little Prince*

Luise went to afterschool, as I didn't finish work until four o'clock.

She was happy there and made all sorts of things in the workshop. Several of her linocuts still adorn the walls of my living room. One print featuring a princess always catches my eye. I love the picture and see Luise whenever I look at it. It warms me. Luise herself didn't think the princess picture was very good. On the whole, she was never completely satisfied with the things she made.

Alfred was the afterschool teacher Luise felt most comfortable with. He did a lot of theater and music with the kids. She enjoyed this, so whenever Alfred was on duty she had a good day. It didn't always go so well when he wasn't at work.

The deputy head, Steen, felt that Luise had a socialization problem. He thought she occasionally had a hard time playing with other children, especially in a group. I knew very well what Steen was talking about. I had also noticed Luise had more fun playing with her friends at home, where she felt secure.

Steen suggested that Luise should get psychiatric help.

Oh no, not again! But we had no choice. Steen informed us that the afterschool center could not be responsible for her if she didn't get help.

From the fall of 1980 Luise spent two afternoons a week in therapy sessions at Copenhagen University's Institute of Psychology. She had both individual and group therapy for three years and I went to the on-site sessions for parents.

There's no doubt in my mind that she was happy during the time she spent there. It was obvious from the way she talked about the staff there. I think she saw it as a sanctuary, which was understandable, as the psychologist and staff all saw her as the wonderful person she was. And she was very aware of that. From the way they talked about her, I felt this was one of the rare times I could say: 'It's Luise they're talking about, not a problem or a diagnosis.'

In our sessions with the psychologists they were always keen to talk about her resources. I loved to spend time with them going through the list of all the things she was good at. I hadn't been involved in this sort of discussion very often.

I remember them asking me one day: 'Have you wondered about Luise's ability to get from one end of the city to the other by public transport while still only seven?' No, I really hadn't thought much about it – that's just the way she was.

But that's right. After taking a taxi to the Institute the first couple of times, she had memorized how to get there by bus, and she insisted on doing this from then on.

Then we started the detective work, and one by one her strengths became clearer. Her knowledge of what was happening in the world around her was at the forefront. Then came her love of art and music and her desire to share this with others. Her ability to cope with problems and situations were also beyond what one would expect of a child her age. She also had a good memory that enabled her to remember what she had learned and experienced. They said she had a photographic memory.

Based on the Institute's observations, the task now was to figure out how we could support Luise going forward, so her interaction with other children could improve.

She also needed help to develop her resources and improve her self-confidence.

I enjoyed these sessions. They gave me the positive energy I needed to cope with everyday life and the sometimes overwhelming cascade of negative talk about Luise. Unfortunately, I also realized that her abilities were not like most people's and therefore may not have counted for much in the eyes of teachers.

I must say that the following description of Luise is sober and the tone is positive.

Institute of Psychology observations from mid-1980 (excerpts):
Luise has difficulty playing with more than one person at a time. When playing with a group, she tends to play off to the side while still remaining part of the larger group. Luise feels good about this type of play. Luise copes best when things happen on her own terms. She has done the Wechsler Intelligence Scale for Children (WISC) test. Test results from the various segments are very uneven. In some areas she achieves results well above her age level, and in others below her age level. But the result indicates basically good intellectual resources. Result of the therapeutic part of the treatment: Luise is a very delicate girl whose anxiety is easily triggered. In situations where she feels under pressure she gets despondent and loses confidence that she can do anything at all. She sometimes gets angry when faced with a task she feels incapable of handling or which she does not understand. Luise has autistic traits but cannot be diagnosed as autistic, since her development was normal over her first year.

Chart notes May 1983 (excerpts):
Luise must still be described as an extremely fragile and delicate girl with a loosely organized personality structure, which is easily overwhelmed by external and internal pressures, causing her to become confused and react angrily. Her manner has a rigid and unyielding edge to it. Her sense of the world around her is somewhat colored by aggression (or aggressive projections). Her conceptual abilities range from the vague and diffuse and sometimes overlapping to the idiosyncratic and autistic. From a diagnostic point of view, Luise occupies a gray area. She has autistic traits but she functions far too well to be autistic. Her intellectual achievements are too advanced for this diagnosis. It seems as if she sometimes does not understand what is being said to her, mostly when it involves long and complicated messages. It is almost as if she gets lost for brief moments. She has very little self-confidence and doesn't believe what she does is good enough. She can become frustrated and angry when she cannot accomplish what is asked of her, especially if demands are made insistently. Luise can seem fumbling and clumsy, and so has a little trouble with the usual children's games involving body movement. For example, she doesn't jump or run very well.

I can clearly recognize Luise in these notes. I had also experienced Luise's short fuse. And, as described, it was when there was a task she couldn't handle or didn't understand. But, like anyone else, she also reacted with anger in situations where she actually was hurt because she felt misunderstood. Her problem was simply that she was misunderstood far more often than normal children because of her lack of 'social skills.' It became increasingly clear to me that Luise also got angry with herself when she could not fulfill the expectations of others or herself. Luise was always unhappy and apologetic about these outbursts afterwards.

Luise, you could at times seem very distracted. I sometimes got a feeling that you were in another world and didn't hear every-

thing that was said to you. In situations where you felt safe you understood very well what others were saying and would respond immediately. Other times when you were unsure, your response would be a jumble of random, unconnected words.

If a respected professor behaved in a similar fashion, it would be interpreted positively as a sign of distractedness. Professors are allowed to be absent-minded, as they have many important thoughts to ponder. But for Luise, it was interpreted as a sign that she simply went missing for brief moments, and sadly not because of weighty musings.

It is clear that Luise falls in a gray area in terms of diagnosis. The observations suggest that Luise has autistic traits. Autism is rejected because she functions too well and her intellectual achievements are too high for this diagnosis. Asperger's syndrome is within the autism spectrum, but the symptoms are not as burdensome and therefore easily overlooked. But the wide divergence in performance levels and the stonewalling – what I've referred to as the nay-saying problem – are typical Asperger's traits. The fumbling and bumbling described above are also common in children with Asperger's syndrome.

Today a lot of attention is paid to children with this diagnosis. But this was not the case in 1992, nor in the 1980s. When Luise should have had this diagnosis, mental health practitioners didn't really know much about Asperger's. It was probably one of the reasons why Luise and many other children became pawns in the psychiatric treatment system. However, this is not even close to being an excuse.

Based on the Institute of Psychology's observations, Luise was referred to the Cerebral Palsy Clinic at the National Hospital. Here the idea was to examine whether Luise's poor motor skills and bodily coordination abilities had an underlying neurological cause. The plan was good and we were optimistic.

9

DETERIORATION

In Denmark we're always finding fault.
We seek out defects and inadequacies in need of repair.
We overlook a person's resources.
And these resources quietly fade.

Luise was referred to the Cerebral Palsy Clinic because of her poor motor skills.

Here she would undergo sensory integration therapy. The purpose of the therapy was to strengthen her motor skills and coordination.

Preliminary investigations began. They studied her coordination, muscle tone, whether she was confused between right and left, and much more. It was based on the knowledge that people lacking motor control also have difficulty concentrating and therefore find it difficult to learn.

Today I can see that the reason we give children with Asperger's syndrome sensory integration training is to help them develop their power of concentration and thereby their ability to learn.

We started sessions at the clinic in July 1983.

Every week we did a small function test following a verbal session. We had many sessions, partly because the different therapists wanted to hear about Luise, partly because new practitioners often came into the picture.

A child must be present while people are talking about her. It's called 'respect for the individual's integrity.' The underlying idea is fine. 'Don't talk about someone unless that person is present, since he or she must be able to comment.' But we were still talking over Luise's head, since the questions posed were very technical and hardly something an 11-year-old child could relate to.

In the sessions I had to describe everything you couldn't do. There was no interest in what you could do.

It must have been awful for you having to sit and listen to your mother, who was supposed to be your rock-solid supporter and defender, repeatedly belittle you like that.

But I didn't know any better then. I really thought it was of crucial importance for your future that I answer all the 'negative' questions. So I resigned myself to the task.

I still think that these many conversations over your head may have meant that you began to doubt my love for you.

I see why you no longer liked me singing 'You are my sunshine, my only sunshine.' How could you believe that I meant what I sang when I was always telling the therapists about how poorly you were doing?

For Luise one consequence was that she began see herself increasingly in terms of all the things her mother said she couldn't do. It wasn't exactly what she needed when she already lacked self-confidence.

For me there was some consolation when all those painful exchanges at the clinic finally led to an extensive and excellent training program, free of verbal sessions.

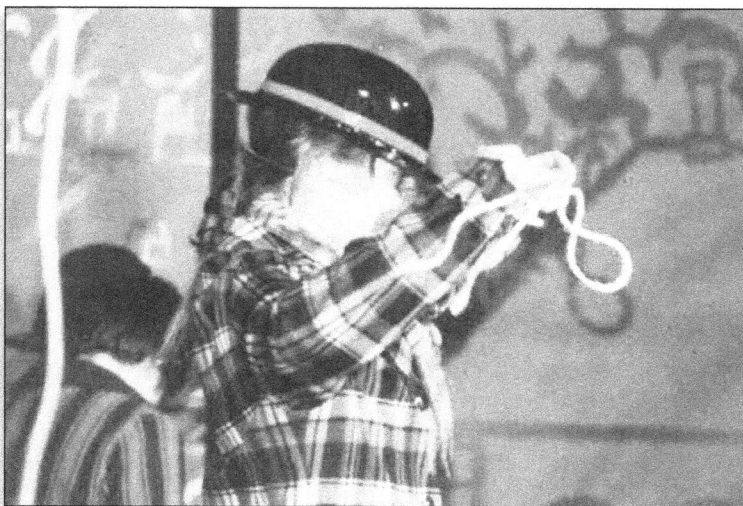

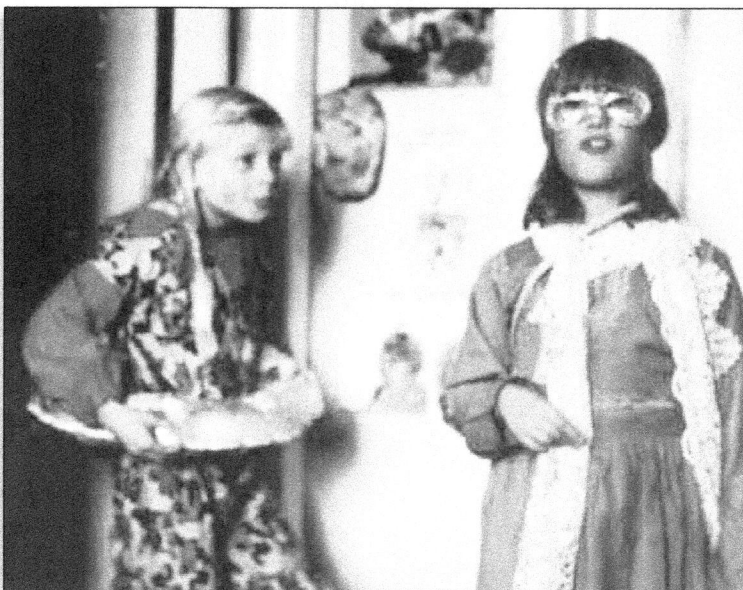

Luise as a clown at Brumleby's 1977 Spring Festival;
on stage with Mille, who became a professional actress

A six-month therapeutic exercise program was also scheduled. Among other things this included structured exercises that were designed as play. There were also various exercise machines you could train on, under strict instructions from a therapist. At our very first training session we learned some exercises/games we could do at home. We were also told it would be a great idea to walk home through Fælledparken, a big city park, marching like soldiers with arms swinging. This was an excellent way to improve coordination between the right and left brain hemispheres, as well as being fun.

Can you remember how much you were looking forward to getting into the program, if for no other reason than to try out the advanced machines?

But the therapeutic exercise program never really got underway. We received no explanation. We were told they had made an appointment for us at the Department of Neurology.

10

NEUROLOGY DEPARTMENT

I sat there week after week and talked about
all the things you couldn't do.
You sat beside me listened to
all the things I said you couldn't do.
Nobody asked you anything.

We were called in for discussions at the National Hospital's Neurology Department, where I again had to sit and tell people about all the things you couldn't handle. Yet another practitioner could now make more chart notes.

From mid-1983 to March 1984, when you were diagnosed with hidden epilepsy, we usually had one session a week.

I hated having to sit and talk about you that way – again. At the same time I was convinced it was important for me to do so. Any data the new neurologist got from me might help them arrive at the right diagnosis. Luise, you should know that I loved you as you were and that I always wished there were more people like you.

It was also dawning on me how important it was for Luise to get diagnosed, so she might get some peace and quiet in her daily life. It was clearly a strain for her, hearing all the discussions where she was always being weighed and measured. One could say that a diagnosis can serve as a form of protection, as there are clear rules for interpreting the behavior of a person who has been 'categorized' – and for how the person should be treated.

After a series of discussions the neurologist arrived at a possible diagnosis. We were told that Luise might have hidden epilepsy, also known as absence seizures or petit mal seizures. It meant that she could be far away for brief moments, without her or anyone around her being aware of it. Perhaps this might explain why she sometimes seemed absent-minded. We heard several case studies of how debilitating hidden epilepsy can be for a child.

I remember how relieved we were on receiving this information. I believe that, in my excitement, I failed to give any thought to the fact that this was a diagnosis focusing on all the things Luise couldn't do, without regard for the areas where she had tested well above her age level in the 1980 WISC test, including intellectual tasks. On the contrary, these strengths did not influence the assumptions behind the new diagnosis.

Nor was there any focus on her autistic traits and poor motor skills.

The neurologist must have been looking for signs of hidden epilepsy. Her questions and our answers just seemed to fit with this disorder.

Epilepsy is normally associated with fits – a person collapses in convulsions and 'goes missing.' Luise had never had fits, but she may have suffered from mental absences.

Since she had no visible signs of epilepsy, the diagnosis had to be confirmed by an electro-encephalogram (EEG) test to measure brain activity.

The EEG test showed a 'faulty oscillation.' We were told this was a sign of epilepsy.

This is how they explained what happens in the brain when you have epilepsy: the condition is caused by obstruction in the brain's highly complex impulse system (transmission system), which may lead to a kind of short-circuiting.

The neurologist described it in such a way that I instinctively came to equate the brain's impulse system with what I knew from school, from physics classes dealing with electrical impulses.

I saw in my mind's eye two electrical wires connected. A poor connection can be the cause of two problems.

Either the system short-circuits – sparks fly and everything goes dark. This corresponded to an epileptic fit.

Alternately, you can also connect the wires wrong and not cause a short circuit – but neither do you get any electrical activity. This corresponded to hidden epilepsy.

Luise showed no visible sign of short-circuiting, but we realized she might have moments without brain activity (absences). And during these moments she didn't really know what had happened. This might be the reason she sometimes didn't understand long-winded instructions.

From a treatment point of view it didn't matter whether there was a short circuit (epileptic seizure) or whether it was simply absence of brain activity (hidden epilepsy). Luise had a 'mechanical malfunction' which could be 'repaired' with medication. Deprakine, a relatively new drug, was suggested.

Wonderful! We got the impression that a little medication would solve her problems, so she could then start a new and normal life.

She was happy to have a plausible explanation for her problems. She was optimistic on hearing that the medication could make her life normal.

I was also happy and relieved to hear this rational and understandable explanation, which made it clear to me that many of the problems she'd had could have been caused by hidden epilepsy.

But could the autistic traits and the very poor motor skills also be cured with this medication?

We trusted the physician's assessment. And overshadowing everything was our hope that her life would get easier.

It never occurred to us that the new diagnosis and the cure for it would prove disastrous for Luise. We had no idea how anti-epileptic medication worked. Our knowledge of medicine was limited largely to the over-the-counter pain-killers, where it didn't make much difference if a person took one or two pills.

The medication effects were to be monitored during a hospital stay in the children's psychiatric ward. In other words, there was a shift from a neurological treatment approach to a psychiatric treatment regimen, though still at the National Hospital.

11

CHILD PSYCHIATRY WARD

Caustic grief hangs like heavy gray fog in my mind.
I cannot find even a moment of peace.
Your sad eyes burrow into my heart, pleading for help.
I cannot ease your torment, though I would gladly pledge my life.
Your carers have reserved the right to help you.
I fear they will help you all the way to hell
in the holy name of science.

Your grieving mother

Don't doctors understand that a mother's worst misery is seeing that her child is not thriving?

Don't they understand a mother will do anything in her power to make her child get better?

Don't they understand a mother's entire life is about her child and all her thoughts and mental energy revolve around what she can do to help her child get better?

Doctors have children too. They must surely know these feelings? They would also do everything in their power to ensure their own children are doing well. I am sure that doctors, like everyone else, are convinced that, as parents, they know their children best, because they have watched them grow from close up.

Why can't health care providers understand that we parents also have a good feel for what is right and wrong for our children – even if they're being treated by a specialist?

You made your serious entry into the mental health care system in the spring of 1984. For you it was a little like going to jail. The heavy doors clanked shut behind you, and there was no way out.

You had to wave goodbye to your peer group in Brumleby. You never really came back to your friends, or your games, or the annual children's theater.

You did come home on weekends, but all the medicine you took left you lethargic and bereft of energy, so you slept most of the time.

It makes me so sad to think that your sheltered childhood ended in March 1984, when at age 11½ you were admitted to the children's psychiatric ward at the National Hospital.

Although the staff there did everything within their power to make life easier for all you young patients, the problem was that you were now thought of as a psychiatric case. I could feel this from the staff on my visits.

As I understood it, Luise was hospitalized because antiepileptic drugs had to be carefully controlled and monitored when prescribed for children. I now know that these drugs dramatically affect the brain's transmission systems. And since a child's brain is not fully developed, extra care must be taken with the medication – indeed, the use of these powerful drugs on children should as far as possible be avoided.

Luise quickly got into the role of psychiatric patient. I noticed this when we first stayed at our newly acquired summer house in Kulhuse in the summer of 1984. The neighbors welcomed us and we talked a little about ourselves. She said: 'My name is Luise. They've put me in the National Hospital, because I'm mentally ill.'

From March 1984 and for many years afterwards, as a helpless bystander I watched Luise zigzag through I don't know how many different treatment approaches, where the caregivers obviously did not work as a team. At the time this was just an impression I got. Today, based on the chart notes I've since obtained, I now see this really was the case.

I'm not suggesting I was the perfect mother, who had a firm grip on the situation and knew what treatment was right for Luise. But I obviously had a sense of whether the various medications and therapies were having a positive or negative effect on my daughter. For example, I was certain that sensory integration training would have been good for Luise. It was written up several times in the chart notes: 'The mother continues to request sensory integration training.'

Luise first started with this therapy in late 1983, but each time her regimen was changed, which happened often, and the therapy was interrupted and then resumed. This meant that she never really managed to get consistent, continuous treatment – or even make a proper start.

I hadn't found any secret formula, far from it. However, I could easily see when the drug treatment was making her worse. But what good was that when her caregivers felt she was getting better? This was what they thought for at least the first year and a half. Later they realized she showed noticeable improvement without the medication.

While in treatment in the children's psychiatric ward Luise came home three days a week. This meant that I could follow her closely when adjusting medication dosage. I gradually began to doubt whether the medication was right for Luise. For example, I saw she was becoming increasingly irascible and fussy.

There wasn't a particular date and time when I realized this was the wrong treatment. It happened gradually, while I was hoping I was mistaken and thinking everything would surely get better with time. For quite some time I accepted the doctor's explanation that Luise was not doing well because she wasn't getting enough medicine. So I indirectly went along with increasing the drug dose.

In December 1984, the doctors at the children's psychiatric ward were of the opinion that Luise was getting the correct medication doses, so she was discharged and came home. We got a card marked with five appointments dates, about once every month. Here we were to follow up on the treatment. Now that Luise was at home around the clock, my suspicions were soon confirmed. The medicine was not helping her – it was actually making her worse.

I had already told the neurologist this at our first follow-up meeting. Then things began to go haywire. My appointments with the neurologist were now being cancelled. Our family doctor suddenly wouldn't let me be present during his talks with Luise. His reasoning was that I had a negative effect on my daughter.

I didn't understand what was happening. I chose to believe that there must have been a misunderstanding. I had previously enjoyed a good working relationship with the care providers, and now everything suddenly turned bad.

I can now see from National Hospital records that by 1985 they had initiated a close working relationship with our family doctor.

It should be a positive sign when a family doctor and a medical institution work together. But in Luise's case it meant that at age 13 she had to speak with the doctor alone, which she absolutely did not like.

The English writer George Orwell in 1948 wrote his speculative novel *1984*. Here he coined the term 'new-speak.'

He used it primarily in a political context, e.g. 'War is peace,' and such. Likewise, he provided a rich selection of prevailing euphemisms, which he believed were used to camouflage morally repugnant ideas and actions.

1984 was the year when Luise optimistically went to the hospital to be treated for 'hidden epilepsy.' It was the year when the foundation was laid for several years of incorrect medical treatment. In short, I can now see it was the year everything turned Orwellian. I could describe her treatment progress in Orwellian terms. She got help, they said. The help

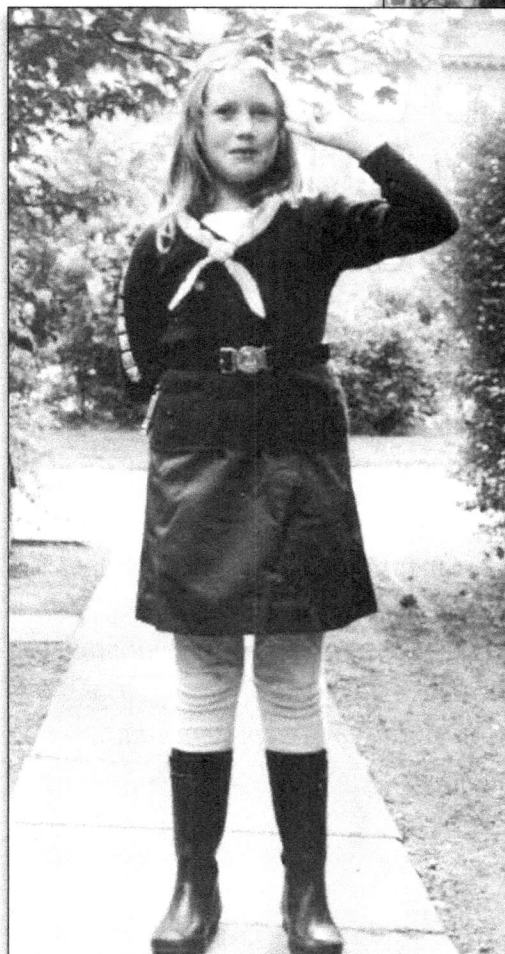

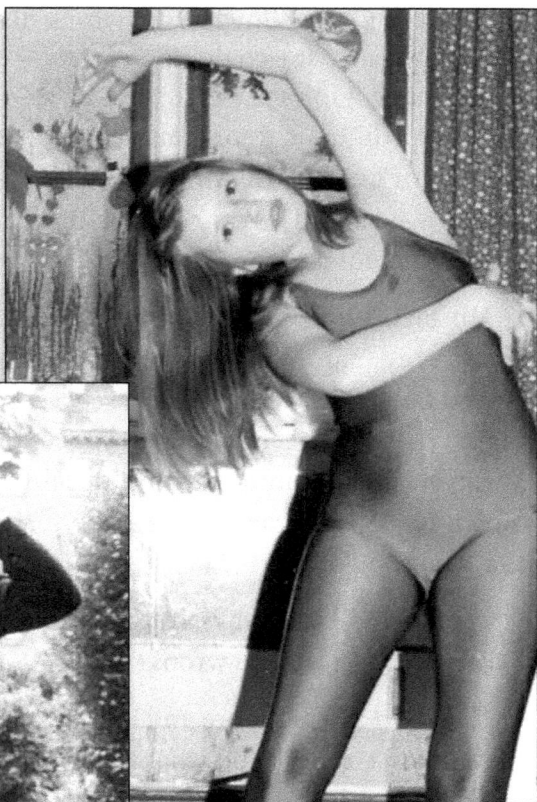

Practicing her jazz ballet moves, and in full Girl Scout uniform.

consisted of their giving her the wrong diagnosis. The diagnosis was a disaster, because she could not tolerate the medication, which caused her permanent injury.

I was still invited for conferences. The providers had to speak with the next of kin of a minor. But the form and content of these sessions had changed after I'd reported that the drugs made Luise worse. It made me feel uncomfortable.

In fact, I was pushed to the sidelines, as 'professional communication' now mainly took place among the specialists, our family doctor and Social Services. I clearly sensed that my concerns about Luise's treatment were perceived as annoyances that obstructed and delayed the caregivers' self-reinforcing procedural certainties. The fact that I had known Luise for her entire life – the very basis for my evaluation – was now irrelevant.

I began to blame myself for this chaos. I had a growing fear that I had caused things to go wrong.

I started talking more and more with friends about Luise's care, because I didn't understand what was going on. Luise couldn't bear to hear my incessant chatter about her treatment and see me constantly leafing through journals and notes about her case. So she chose to act.

One day I came home to find that the folder where I kept all the records and letters was gaping open and empty. I asked what had happened to the contents, and you replied: 'It got thrown away.' I took the hint that it was time for me to relax my interminable focus on your treatment. Whether it was right or wrong, it polluted your life. So I swallowed my irritation and pretended it was OK that you'd thrown out the papers.

12

IF I HAD A MILLION

If I had a million, I'd find a good place
where Luise would be allowed
to develop at her own pace.
A place where Luise wouldn't always
be molded from a template

'If I had a million.' This was a phrase I always used when teaching Danish as a second language as an example of the grammatical verb mood called the subjunctive. I used it as a model to explain that when you start a sentence with 'if' and, as in English, use the past tense, it changes the meaning – so you actually don't have a million!

I've often thought that if I had a million I'd find a good place for Luise and me, where she would get to live and grow at her own pace.

When we spent a vacation on the Spanish island of Formentera in the summer of 1980, we met a Danish woman. She had moved to Formentera so her son could grow up without constant intervention from the educational system. Her son had been diagnosed with ADHD. Entangled in the treatment machinery, he was deteriorating rapidly, as she could clearly see. She had money, so she could choose this as an alternative. I admired her for her decision and only wished I could do the same. But we lived on a teacher's salary, which wouldn't get us very far.

One option open to us was a visit to some friends of ours, Elisabeth and her boys Rolf and Oliver, who also lived on Formentera. And it turned out great.

We arrived on the island by ferry early one morning. Rolf and Oliver were standing on the quay. They didn't recognize us because our faces were covered in mosquito bites. We all found it very amusing.

Our friends had a beautiful but primitive house on loan for the summer. It was built of solid stone. Everything in the house was made of stone: bookshelves, cabinet shelves, bedding, etc. We had to fetch water from a well in the yard.

We were on Formentera for a month. Elisabeth and I really got into relaxing. We eventually got so de-stressed that our essential daily chore of drawing water from the well was starting to take all day.

In stark contrast, you children frolicked in the exciting, unfamiliar surroundings far from swings and climbing frames and hovering teachers. There were many playmates your age on the island. Some days you were all so absorbed in your exciting projects that we only saw you at mealtimes. I recall that Elisabeth and I always kept a tub of water outside, warming in the sun, in case you came home covered from head to toe in the powdery dust.

Luise, on Formentera you did great. Nobody here was insisting that you become a group-oriented person, as expected of you in kindergarten. You played well with the other kids. You really didn't run into any conflicts on Formentera. That doesn't mean you didn't say no. But there were no teachers around to make a big deal out of it. If you refused to perform a task, there was usually someone else who stepped up. No problems arose, because you didn't get into situations where you felt under pressure.

You were never teased, as I recall. Anyway, you always talked about wishing we could move to Formentera.

13

THE CONDITION WORSENS

In a bureaucracy, moral concerns of the functionary
are drawn back from focusing on the plight of the objects of action.
They are forcefully shifted in another direction – the job to be done
and the excellence with which it is performed.
It does not matter that much how the 'targets' of action feel or fare.
It does matter, however, how smartly and effectively the actor fulfills
whatever he has been told to fulfill by his superiors.

Zygmunt Bauman, *Modernity and the Holocaust*

As mentioned, Luise's treatment was concluded and she was discharged from the children's psychiatric ward at the end of 1984. She was
to remain at home, on the medication dose that had been judged right
for her. This was 1200 mg of Deprakine daily.

According to the neurologist and the psychiatrist, Luise had benefited from Deprakine. I could see, however, that the medication had
made her distinctly worse. Unhappily, Luise herself could feel that she'd
changed. She often mentioned that she felt she was becoming strange. It
made her feel embarrassed, so she isolated herself even more from her
peers than she had done before going into treatment.

This meant that nine months in the children's psychiatric ward,
with environmental therapy and epilepsy medication, had not remedied
such 'dysfunctions' as stubbornness and lack of social skills. Rather, the
treatment had significantly exacerbated the very symptoms that led to
Luise's initial referral for treatment. The bad news was that she'd also
become quick-tempered and aggressive. Not much was needed before
Luise exploded. It wasn't just Luise and I who saw that the medication

had changed her. I now know that the psychologist from the children's psychiatric ward had observed the same.

This is evidenced in a letter from him to the Institute of Psychology dated May 29, 1984: 'Luise is still odd and she still has her peculiarities, which have become more pronounced after medication.' So the psychologist, who had frequent conversations with Luise, observed that Luise's 'peculiarities' became more pronounced as the medication dosage was increased.

Something is not right here. Luise could not have got significantly better on the drug if her eccentricities were becoming more evident with increased dosages. It was these idiosyncrasies that initially got her into treatment.

A few months after Luise's death I found some of the chart notes and papers I thought she had thrown away years before. They included charts from the National Hospital between 1983 and 1988.

I found them among Luise's old schoolbooks as I was going through the things she'd left.

It took forever to read through the medical records. It was painful.

With the papers in front of me, I tried to get a picture of the process and seek an explanation for some of the incomprehensible things that happened from early 1985 to October 1986.

The neurologist and I started having lots of difficulty working together in early 1985. Shortly after Luise came home from the children's psychiatric ward, the neurologist suddenly seemed dismissive and stressed out. She canceled our appointments. I didn't understand what was happening. It obviously made me very insecure.

It's clear from the record that I was systematically being set up to get cut loose. This was happening in conjunction with my growing fear that the anti-epileptic medication might not be the wonder cure for my daughter.

As I was sure the drug was wrong for Luise, the providers suggested I had taken leave of my senses. They insinuated that I was the reason Luise was not getting better and could not evaluate objectively, since I was not doing that well myself.

Through their 'creative chart notes' the doctors could justify that they cancelled meetings and increased Luise's medication to much too high a level by writing that the drug improved her condition.

This can be seen in the seven chart notes written by the child neurologist in Luise's journal in the spring of 1985. Below I only refer to the portion of each note that leads toward terminating any cooperation with me.

The notes' content is incorrect, and so are the dates. Why is this?

I phoned the neurologist on February 5 1985, according to my correspondence with Social Services. I made contact because Luise had become numb in her arms and legs. I was told that I should immediately start phasing out Deprakine, as this reaction might be a sign of incipient drug poisoning. Luise was to have the dosage reduced by 300 mg every month. This meant she would be drug-free by the beginning of May.

The dosage reduction because of possible overmedication is not mentioned in the chart notes. Excerpts follow:

1. February 13 1985 (a week after we started reducing Luise's drug dose because of the possible onset of drug poisoning): *'According to the mother, Luise faces no problems in daily life.'* Later in the record, it is noted: *'Luise is doing well and we will try raising the Deprakine dosage to 1500 mg.'*

2. March 13 1985: *'The mother phones and tells us that Luise is having a hard time. She is numb in her arms and legs. For this reason the mother has herself reduced the drug dosage. The mother vents that we must completely stop treatment with Deprakine, which I* (i.e. the neurologist) *think is a bad idea.'*

3. April 23 1985: *'The mother rings. She thinks Luise is feeling ad-*

verse effects and cannot tolerate so much medication and should have the dosage reduced. This surprised me somewhat, as it is quite clear we have witnessed a dramatic improvement in behavior since we started the anti-epileptic treatment.'

4. April 26 1985: *'Luise is admitted to the adolescent psychiatric ward at Bispebjerg Hospital. The mother gives the clear impression that she is extremely ambivalent about the medication and the treatment, which was also my impression* (i.e. the neurologist at the National Hospital). *We agree to increase Luise's Deprakine dose.'*

5. May 22 1985: *'The mother is having a very hard time. Luise is doing very well. We* (i.e. the neurologist and psychiatrist at Bispebjerg Hospital) *agree there is no need for further conferences with the mother.'*

6. June 7 1985: *'Luise says she has been hospitalized with something wrong with her stomach. There might be something to this. We're probably not getting complete information from the mother.'*

7. June 17 1985: *'Phone call from the adolescent psychiatric ward. We arrange for the adolescent psychiatric ward to take primary charge of Luise. This is the most appropriate move, so that the mother cannot manipulate the undersigned against the ward, or vice versa.'*

These seven chart note entries don't hold much water. Note 1 says that Luise is doing well and they were trying a dosage increase to 1500 mg. But Luise had started on a reduced dose a week before February 13, when the note was written.

Note 2 describes the telephone conversation, which took place five weeks earlier (!), in which the neurologist said Luise's dosage should immediately be reduced to avoid a possible drug overdose. So on March 13 Luise's dose was down to 600 mg. Later we can see they increased the dose to 900 mg at Solvang in early April. It was this increase I phoned about to question the neurologist on April 23. The dramatic improvement in behavior described in the same chart note was clearly no more dramatic than when they requested a bed in a treatment home in November 1984 for Luise, arguing that she would be too much for me to handle around the clock. Luise first became aggressive and testy after she had started the medication. Before the hospitalization Luise and I had no problems at home, and she was referred to a psychologist because the afterschool center believed she lacked 'social skills' and not because she and I had problems day to day.

According to the experts Luise's condition had not taken a turn for the worse because of the anti-epileptic medication errors. No! Their opinion was that the deterioration was due to hidden epilepsy, which was why she needed more medicine.

In a short space of time Luise had put on an extra 55 lbs. The weight gain happened so fast that the skin on her stomach and thighs cracked open. According to the chart she had only gained 13 lbs.

The seven chart entries illustrate Zygmunt Bauman's claim that functionaries' thinking is not concerned with the target group's condition, or how the 'objects' of their actions are faring, but with how efficiently and skillfully tasks are completed. It seemed like an efficient solution, of course, since there's plenty written about it in the chart. But, unless you already know what was going on, you can't see that what is recorded is incorrect.

My sense that the otherwise excellent cooperation with the neurologist ended when I reported that the medication was in no way good for Luise turned out to be correct. But why did I get shunted to the sidelines?

In reality we were both deeply saddened to see that the treatment we had hoped would help Luise had actually made her worse than ever.

There was nothing we could do, because the neurologist and psychiatrist said that she had clearly benefited from the medicine. When two medical experts make this kind of statement, it becomes an incontrovertible truth. Even though the psychologist who worked with the Institute for Psychology – and thus knew Luise's situation – said the opposite.

Let me break the chronology for a brief comment to illustrate this 'scientific infallibility.'

On November 10, 1986, a new neurologist wrote, after several conferences with Luise: 'As stated, Luise is no longer receiving anti-epileptic treatment. Her condition improved considerably afterwards.'

This was written over a year after the previous neurologist wrote that Luise had got dramatically better on the heavy dose of Deprakine.

Luise indeed felt better after she'd stopped taking the drug. Her explosive, aggressive fits had stopped. She had become more 'normal' but at the same was experiencing serious and debilitating side-effects.

14

'BEST' TREATMENT HOME

*Once effectively dehumanized and hence cancelled
as potential subjects of moral demands,
human objects of bureaucratic task-performance
are viewed with ethical indifference ...
Dehumanized objects cannot have a 'cause',
much less a 'just cause'. They have no 'interests'
to be considered, indeed no claim to subjectivity.*

Zygmunt Bauman, *Modernity and the Holocaust*

We were asked to come in for a conference at the children's psychiatry ward on March 7, 1985.

At the meeting you were told they had found a good place for you to stay awhile. I clearly remember that they gave the impression this was the best place for you. You've often since told me with a wry smile: 'Mom, do you remember that time the psychiatry ward found the best place for me? That was a good one!' You said this with your light-hearted gallows humor. You were good at putting a positive spin on things, turning bad experiences into 'grotesque incidents' – at least, when you'd distanced yourself sufficiently.

The place was called Solvang.

Of course, they could rightly claim it was the best – it was the only treatment center in the Copenhagen metro area.

I don't remember the psychiatrist's exact words, but it was made to sound as if I couldn't have Luise at home anymore, so the psychiatry department had found a really good place where she could stay awhile. This left me speechless. We'd talked about several different kinds of help and support for when Luise came home. We had discussed a possible stay at a treatment center called Nebsmøllegaard, which we both knew because my aunt was a psychological consultant there. But otherwise we'd only talked about support in the home.

So the Solvang idea came as a complete surprise to us both. Luise didn't give the impression that she was unhappy or hurt by the decision. But later I often got it thrown in my face when she was mad at me: 'You never liked me. You've always wanted to get rid of me. I was only eleven years old when you first sent me away.'

But why would they now send Luise to a psychiatric treatment center? She was hospitalized in the psychiatric ward so they could administer the anti-epileptic medication, not because she was a psychiatric case in need of further treatment.

I must admit I had a creepy feeling that I shouldn't oppose the doctor's recommended course of action. Now that I have the papers from Social Services I can see I was right to feel suspicious. I came across a letter from the children's psychiatry ward, dated six months earlier, seeking a place in a treatment center on the grounds that Luise was a very difficult educational challenge 24 hours a day.

You must know that I didn't think of you as a difficult educational challenge. You were my beautiful daughter and we did fine in our daily life.

I'd never given any indication that I couldn't have you at home. Quite the contrary.

You were to start on March 18, 1985, a week after we were informed of the move.

We visited Solvang a few days later.

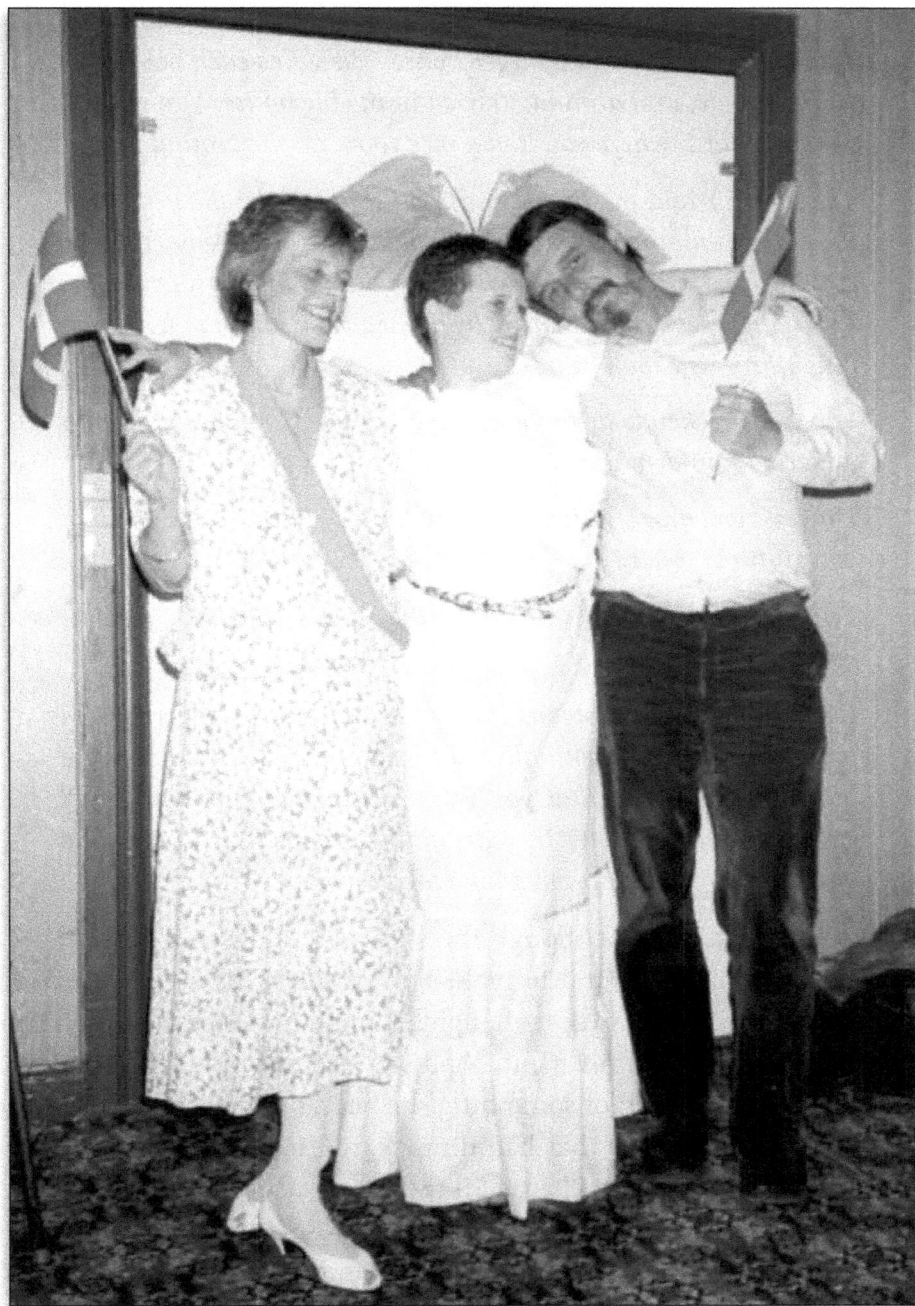

Celebrating confirmation day with Mom and Dad.

We got a good first impression of the place. The institution con-sisted of two villas and a larger house. The villas each housed 12 young people, and around 20 lived in the big house. You were to stay in Villa 1, where you had a nice room on the ground floor.

The director told me that you should think of the place as your new home and that we parents should take an active part in our children's new life, come on visits and attend the various events. I was always welcome to drop by at mealtimes and eat with you. This was music to my ears.

You had weekends at home every other week. We were given a folder with information about the place.

Do you remember, Luise, you were kind of happy at the idea of your future home?

I often dropped by to visit you in the Villa in the early days. It was quite pleasant.

But it soon became obvious I wasn't as welcome as advertised in the literature. You eventually said I shouldn't visit you, because the staff teased you that you were missing your mother (good heavens, you were only 12 years old!). I stopped my dinnertime visits. Our good first impression faded away.

It almost seemed as though the staff were harassing Luise. They explained to me they did it to make her 'strong.' This was in contrast to all the permissiveness they thought I practiced. Luise was often the cause of 'collective punishment.' And she still ended up in situations where she was accused of something she hadn't done. I remember the case of a ghetto blaster that had disappeared from a room. The staff reported that they had gathered all the young people together to find out who had 'taken' the radio. In their opinion Luise obviously had a guilty conscience, since she couldn't explain herself properly. She was therefore declared the culprit. When Luise 'didn't want to' tell what had happened, they had to punish everyone. Luise was therefore to blame that her fellow students didn't have a fun evening. Whenever this sort of thing happened, she was in the doghouse.

All the same, you were very well liked by your peers because of your physical strength and sense of humor, which made people feel calm and secure. I don't know how to describe it. But it must be the same kind of human strength that can calm animals. One time you stopped a runaway horse in Kulhuse. Our neighbor's little three-year-old, Rune, was in the road in front of our summer house. In the distance we could hear a horse galloping towards us. You rushed into the road, grabbed Rune and got him into the garden, and then walked up to the runaway horse, which thankfully stopped. You stroked the horse's head and talked to it soothingly. I was terrified and could barely grasp what had happened.

It may have been this calmness, along with your humor, courage and love of adventure that encouraged several youngsters to seek your companionship.

It was only later that I heard the story about Luise and Rasmus's field trip to our summer house in Kulhuse. Rasmus was 15 and always getting into trouble. They went to Kulhuse to visit our newly acquired cottage, but Luise had forgotten to take into account that it was dark at 4 o'clock in winter. There was no street lighting around the summer houses, so they couldn't see a thing and couldn't find the cottage.

They got lucky and were given a ride by a couple who lived on a big farm near Frederikssund. Luise later told me they were treated like earls and dukes. The poor wretches were given a nice hot bath. After their bath they were served good food and invited to stay for the night. Luise described the place as if it were a stately home.

Your absence was not reported. That could be because the staff didn't realize you were gone until the following day, when they got a phone call from the couple.

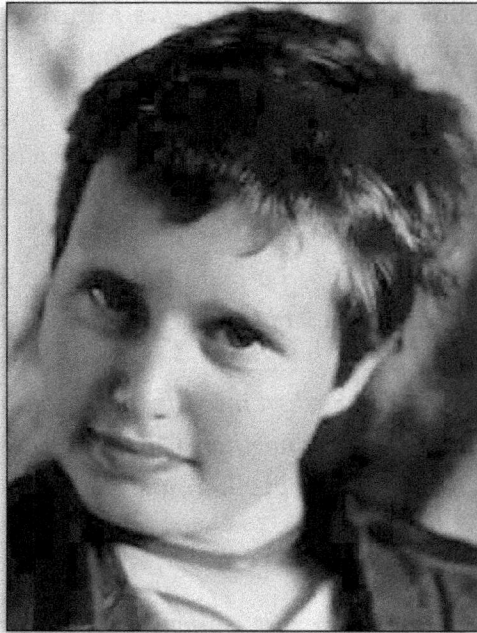

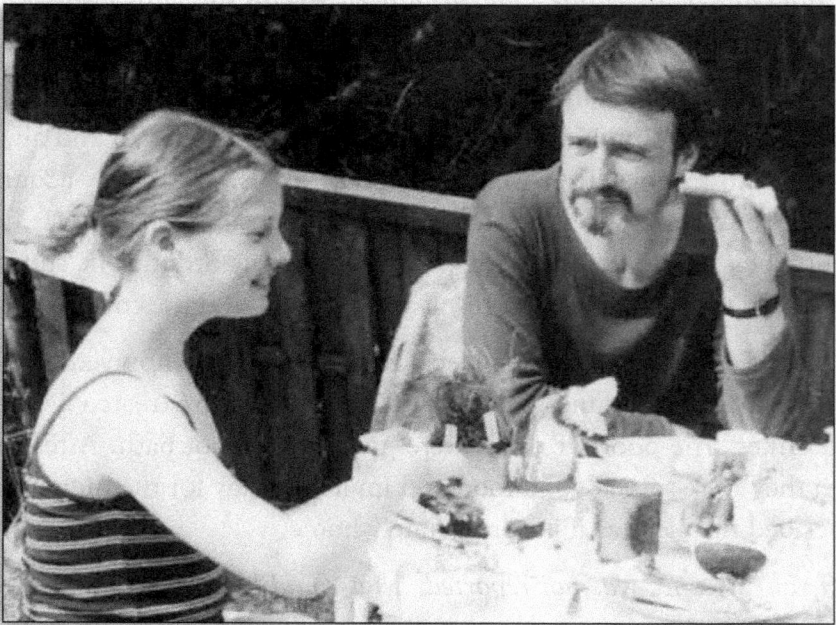

Lunch with Dad at the summer house.

I must say, however, that the center's director was not reticent in his reporting. You'd only been at the treatment center seven days when you were first reported to the authorities. He noted that the staff had been forced to grab you by the arms to 'correct' you – all for your own good.

One time Luise came home with an arm that was yellow and purple and swollen. Luise said that I needn't do anything about it, as she'd already spoken to the director about it. I called the institution to inquire about details of an upcoming parent conference and was immediately put through to the director, who told me that Luise had made a false report about mistreatment from staff members. I told him about Luise's bruises. His response was that he would submit a report from me also. He indicated that they took these cases very seriously.

I duly received a letter from the care home's director, all very correct and officious. It began: 'We had a minor problem with Luise, which made it necessary for two of our female staff to take hold of Luise by the arm and lead her down to the communal room. When they got to the stairs it was actually necessary to lift her.' The letter continued with a few words about the director's meeting with Luise, who reported she was really mad at the two staff members – though she was smiling while she said this. Then came the explanation that when force is used on a patient the incident must be reported to Social Services, who would decide whether it was a necessary and permissible use of force. The director claimed that it was.

Ten days later, three men from the county offices showed up and interrogated Luise about the bruises.

The result of this interview was that she 'confessed' she had inflicted the blue marks on herself so she could report on a staff member.

Obviously you hadn't purposely bruised yourself on the underside of your upper arm. It was simply technically impossible. But the county officials presumably chose to overlook this fact.

*This meant they didn't have to decide whether there had been
any use of force beyond what was permitted in an institution
under their supervision.*

I sent a request to the Health and Social Services Administration to
view the three reports I was told had been filed about the 'blue marks.'
My request came to nothing, because they unfortunately couldn't find
the reports.

*You never brought up the assault again. You didn't want to be
subjected to a humiliating interrogation where you would still
get the blame.*

*Do you remember the time you were on penicillin? You said it
was to treat a vaginal inflammation. The director told me you
had a throat infection. The two explanations did not tally, so I
called the doctor who had prescribed the penicillin. He wouldn't
discuss it, saying I should call the residential home to get an explanation. But I'd already tried that.*

*Our family doctor could see that you had an infection, which he
suspected had been sexually transmitted.*

You would not tell our doctor what had happened.

*You reacted in a hostile manner when I tried to raise the issue. I was
told never to mention anything about your infection to anyone.*

*It wasn't until several years later you first told of the two older
boys who sometimes came into your room when you were asleep.
One held a pillow over your face while the other went to work on
you. Why didn't you report the assaults to staff members? Was it
out of your fear of another interrogation by county officials?*

*My aunt sat in on a meeting with me at the psychiatric treatment
home in June 1986.*

*It became clear to her at the meeting that we had to get you
out of there.*

After that unpleasant meeting we just wanted to drop by to say goodbye to you in the living room where you were all hanging out. We walked right into another unpleasant performance.

We heard you tell a staff member: 'I have a headache.' She replied, 'Do you have a headache? What fun!' She then addressed your fellow inmates in a mocking tone: 'Did you hear – Luise has a headache. Just think, Luise has a headache, isn't that funny? What should we do about it?' Then the staff and residents laughed at you. You left the room.

After observing this scene, my aunt supported me in getting you out of there as quickly as possible. But it had to be carefully planned because, as she said: 'If you just say you want Luise at home, you run the risk that Social Services might arrange an involuntary confinement.'

There were, of course, all sorts of reports at Social Services about how happy Luise was staying there – and what a 'harmful' mother I basically was.

15

EPILEPSY: WRONG DIAGNOSIS

*Many children and adults
originally diagnosed with epilepsy
and given drug treatment for the illness
do not, in fact, have epilepsy.*

Jyllands-Posten newspaper

As so often before, I found that I was cut off when I started questioning whether the treatment Luise was receiving was right for her.

I was made to appear suspect and was unjustly accused of obstructing the treatment. I sensed that the providers almost blamed me for the fact that she was not improving. I had no idea what to do or where to turn for help.

My friends were getting tired of hearing about my problems, which were fast becoming theirs.

As mentioned, I learned on February 5 that her drug dosage would be reduced when I called to report she felt numbness in her body.

She was down to 600 mg when she started at the residential care home.

At Solvang they immediately increased the Deprakine dosage again.

Naturally I was sure there had been a misunderstanding and phoned the neurologist at the National Hospital. As detailed in Chapter 13, this was when I could suddenly never get hold of her. I can now see that I'd been excluded and that, without my knowledge, treatment had been transferred to Bispebjerg Hospital's adolescent psychiatric ward.

The treatment center advertised their effective problem-solving by their frequent reports to the Social Security and Health Administration and local collaborating agencies. If the volume of reports were the yardstick, they would be doing an excellent job solving the problem.

The reports painted a very negative picture of Luise and me. Luise was untruthful and manipulative. She cheated and deceived people. She banged her head against the wall, as mentioned in a letter dated March 25, 1985. This was seen as a sign of my spoiling her, the report said. But it was actually the result of her powerlessness and desperation.

I reportedly had a very negative influence on my daughter, which made it difficult for teachers to get her on a steady footing. For example, I once let her stay home under the 'pretext' that she was ill. According to a report the care home sent to Social Services, she hadn't been sick at all but, as Luise told them, the two of us had been running around town, visiting Tivoli (the popular city center amusement park) and Flakfortet (an old sea fortress in the Sound). The care home never called me to confirm Luise's colorful account, which of course had no bearing on what had actually happened.

Luise indeed was very ill all that week. She had actually had a nervous breakdown and had tried to take her own life, because she didn't want to go back to the institution. Our doctor said she should stay home for at least a week and that we should try to find another place for her.

Her breakdown occurred about three months after she'd moved into the new residential care home.

I received a follow-up letter from the care home director a few days later, full of complaints about Luise's obstructive behavior and her alleged refusal to accept help from the staff. She had complained for four days about stomach pains, but they had failed to deal with this, claiming she had normal bowel movements.

The next day, the Easter half-term break began. Now we could look forward to eight wonderful free days at home in Brumleby. I took the bus to pick you up, as usual. You could hardly walk. You were sick and doubled up with constipation.

You told me that staff members wouldn't let you sit in peace on the toilet, but unlocked the door and let kids and staff stand and laugh at you while you sat and tried to take care of business.

I called the hospital emergency. You were immediately admitted to the National Hospital.

You had bad constipation. I got a severe reprimand for waiting so long before we reported the condition. But your stomach problem had obviously been building up for some time.

Here's an extract from the National Hospital's discharge report, dated April 3, 1985: 'Twelve-year-old girl hospitalized for suspected acute appendicitis. Symptoms emerged approx. 10 days before. Severe pain. On examination, the colon feels full. If the patient gets constipation again, she must be readmitted for flushing with Mannitol *(a mild children's laxative)*.'

The home's assertion that you didn't have constipation but were eliminating normally was incorrect.

Your 'diminished sense of reality' has been described in many reports to Social Services, as in the following letter. This was the third letter sent to Social Services in less than three weeks after you started residential treatment.

Letter dated April 5 1985.
'Dear Mrs. Christensen,
It is very difficult for us to deal with Luise. She has no sense of reality. I do not know how we can tackle the following problem. As we sit and watch television, Luise suddenly says: 'I know them. I've visited them in Palestine. It was very difficult to visit them because there were police everywhere.' It happens repeatedly that she says she knows

someone from the TV, and then her imagination runs away with her as she tells incredible stories. She also believes she saw herself on TV in Blågårds Square. She also says she knows Troels Trier (a well-known Danish musician and artist). When we try to correct her and tell her that it is only TV and she has not been there, she gets moody and will not talk to us anymore. She goes to bed soon afterwards. It is unbelievable that she lives in such an unhealthy fantasy world.'

The letter went on to give several examples of people on TV you said you knew or places you had been. These were seen as products of your pathological fantasy world.

But everything you told them was true.

Luise, you were shot down because your statements were promptly rejected with an instruction that you mustn't lie. They told me that you connected yourself with celebrities on TV because you were very sick. The staff had many elaborate explanations of where your penchant for lying might lead in later life.

Your stories didn't come from a sick fantasy world, however.

We were in Palestine in 1981. Four of us went. The purpose of the trip was to interview several Palestinians, including the mayor of Nablus, Basham Shaaka, who had lost his leg in a car bomb attack.

I saw a segment on Basham Shaaka and the car bombing in a documentary on Palestine on Danish TV. I assume it was the same program you were viewing at the treatment home when you said, 'I know them. I've visited them in Palestine.' You could have shown the staff and residents the photographs we had taken of the Shaaka family on our trip, but you gave up, as they obviously didn't believe you. You were hurt and sulking and went to bed, as it says in the letter they sent to Social Services.

You were completely in your element when we visited foreign parts.

Your ability to communicate in foreign languages was remarkable. It meant that we could easily make contact with the local population.

One of many people you engaged with in Palestine was Hussein, who had a leather shop. Hussein was very happy to have you around. He gave you everything you pointed to. I recently found a leather purse, a toy camel and other small gifts from him. Hussein tried to teach you Arabic, and you were willing to learn. Hussein and his friends laughed a lot at your pronunciation. Your eagerness to achieve perfect pronunciation sometimes produced hilarious results. You were so aware of the frequency of the voiced 'z' sound in Arabic that you overused it. This had you saying 'titty' (biz in Arabic) when you wanted to say 'cat' (bis in Arabic). Your misplaced voiced sibilant raised our spirits, and we had no problem communicating. Hussein's apartment was located in the Palestinian market, the souk. We felt the presence of history as we sat and ate dinner in his home, a curve-shaped room where you could only stand up in the middle and where the curved stone walls bore evidence of origins well over a thousand years ago. Strange inscriptions dotted the ancient walls. We felt transported to the days when Jesus walked in Jerusalem. There was no kitchen in the dwelling, so dinner was brought from the nearest food vendor.

We were excited by the food. We soon fell in love with baklava, their sweet pastry.

Our visit to Mayor Basham Shaaka lasted two days. We stayed with his family and you played with his two girls. As you had told them at the care home, there was a police guard outside the house during our visit. They were a constant presence, as the family was under house arrest.

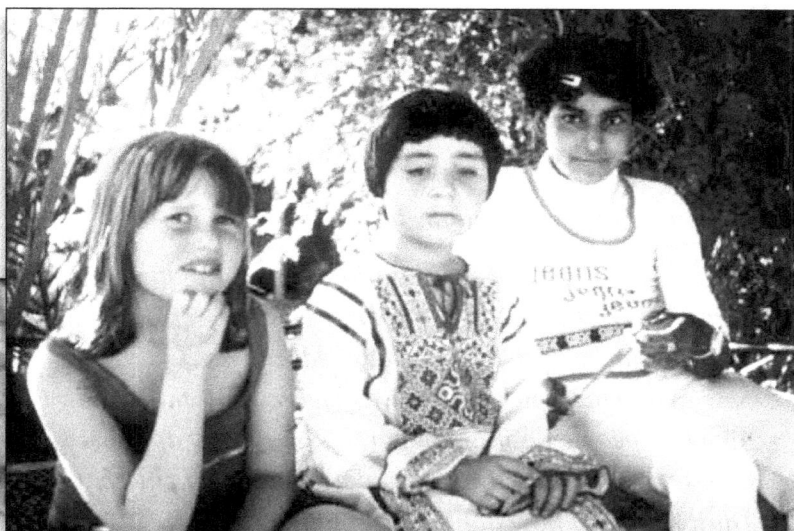

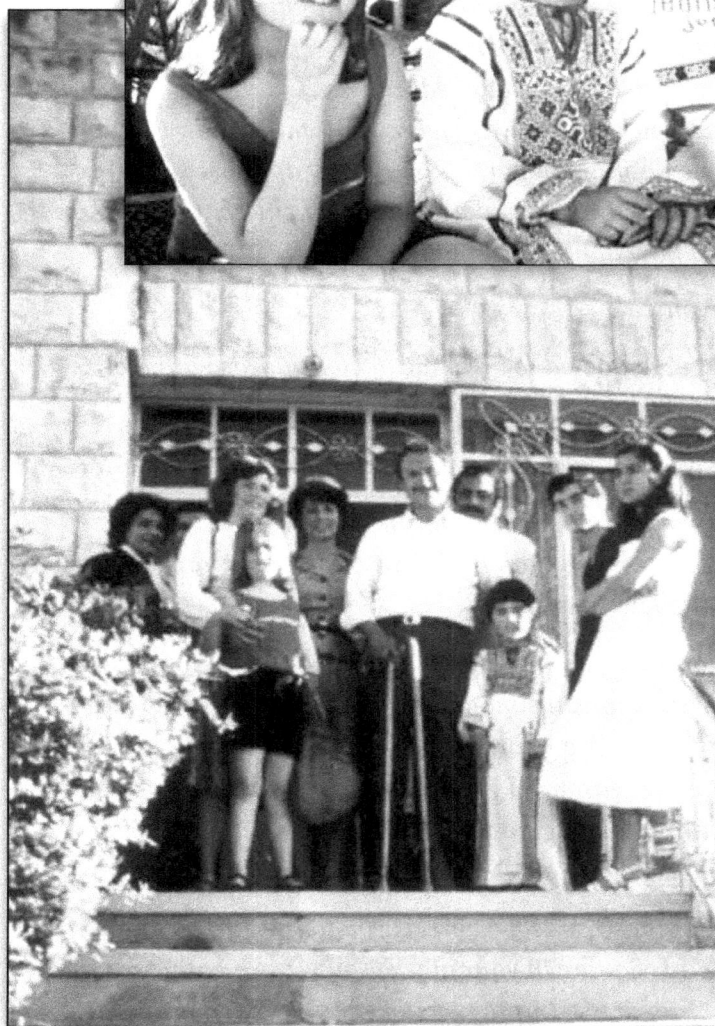

Luise visiting the mayor's family in Nablus, Palestine.

Westerners visiting the mayor were always seen as a problem by the Israeli guards.

They duly took our passports and darkly hinted we might not get them back.

It could mean a prison for us.

But you took care of the situation as we said our goodbyes to the mayor and his family. You ran over to the grim-looking guards toting machine guns. You laughed and said 'Shalom', chatting away in what you thought was Hebrew, all the while gesticulating like people do in these parts. The guards apparently couldn't resist you, so we got our passports back. Fortunately, you never quite realized how dangerous it all was.

Or perhaps you did?

Because you remembered to greet the armed guards with the Hebrew 'Shalom' instead of the Arabic 'Salaam a leikum'.

This tells me you had a feeling the situation was not trouble-free.

Usually you would randomly throw these greetings around, often in the wrong places – Shalom in the Arab territories and Salaam a leikum in the Jewish areas.

Your assertion that you knew Basham Shaaka was no sick fantasy. It wasn't just in your imagination that you'd been to Palestine and seen the police guard around the mayor's house. Actually, you were the reason we got out of there in good shape, after you charmed the tough guards with your Shalom and Hebrew-sounding gobbledygook.

You also saw yourself on television, as you told them. You danced around Blågårds Square in your mask. You were only three at the time. Each of us dressed up as one of the prominent American politicians we loved to hate. We were taking part in happening instigated by Røde Mor ('Red Mother,' Troels Trier's music/art collective). We all danced in a circle to one of their songs. And we did know Troels Trier. The stories you told at the treatment home were not the product of an imaginary world or a morbid tendency to identify with celebrities.

After a brief stay at Bispebjerg Hospital's adolescent psychiatry ward, the discharge note dated June 18, 1985, said you had become borderline psychotic. But the anti-epileptic drug treatment continued uninterrupted.

16

Doing my best as a mother?

The web tightened.
I ran from pillar to post.
No one could help.
And certainly not your case worker.
We had to continue submitting to
the bureaucratic treatment assumptions.

Luise, you have no idea how much it pained me to watch how you were treated. You had ended up in an institution where the caregivers couldn't find any positive traits in you, and so treated you accordingly. I saw how they used your vulnerabilities, your autistic tendencies, to manipulate you.

I ran from pillar to post hoping to find help. I was afraid that the residential treatment center had a long-term plan built around all their reports to Social Services. I feared they were setting you up to be forcibly institutionalized.

What was happening became ever more incomprehensible to me.

Our family doctor at the time, who previously believed we should get you out of Solvang, suddenly changed his mind. I have since learned that this was because he'd started collaborating with the psychiatrists.

I tried to get help from the Mothers' Support Service. I talked with both a psychologist and a lawyer. This only stoked my fear. The psychologist told me that any action I might take would only make them treat you even worse – a form of municipal punishment for daring to question the authority of their institutions.

The attorney was more direct: 'For God's sake, don't complain about Luise's treatment. I can see there are three serious things you could complain about, but I myself have dealt with Social Services and seen the results parents get when they complain, and it's not encouraging. I'm embarrassed to say it. But it's a fact.'

My aunt had said the same thing.

All my so-called helpers advised me to get the institution to discharge you, which would improve our 'case' somewhat, meaning you couldn't then be legally committed as a psychiatric case.

I went to Social Services in the hope that they would see their treatment center wasn't appropriate for you. I brought along Solvang's letters plus documentation that proved their reports were incorrect, such as their letter to Social Services claiming you lied about being constipated and the discharge report from the National Hospital describing your constipation.

They gave me coffee and excellent pastries at the Social Services office, but the correspondence from Solvang had conveniently vanished. So unfortunately they could not discuss the matter with me. They wouldn't even look at the documents I had brought, which of course were copies of this missing correspondence.

It was not the first or last time I was told that important correspondence to city authorities had handily gone missing.

I had a distinct feeling that the paperwork had not just disappeared.

The cream cakes were really nice. The official was affable and polite. But I left empty-handed.

The web tightened from all sides. I tried to find a new school for you, approaching many of the small independent schools. When they heard that you were in the child psychiatry ward, no school dared 'take responsibility for teaching you,' as they so delicately put it. The afterschool centers said the same. It was very disheartening. How could this be?

I tried and tried but every time ran into an invisible brick wall.

I couldn't tell you any of this, Luise. It would have made you even more insecure. I had to choose the least of all the evils. I just had to be there for you as much as possible.

Solvang began to act as if you were forcibly confined. This meant I rarely got to visit you.

I couldn't talk to your teachers and wasn't allowed to attend school events.

I wrote a letter to the school asking if I could take part in events along with the other parents.

This was the reply (abbreviated):

September 9, 1986
Dear Mrs. Christensen,
Thank you for your letter of August 28. I think it's positive that you are interested in Luise's schooling and would like to have as much contact as possible. We totally agree that home/school collaboration is very important, and this has always worked well with Solvang, which is currently Luise's home. In the interests of our students, it is very important to us that we talk to the same collaborator every time, so the connections between school and home are clear and unambiguous, and this school firmly believes that Solvang meets that need very well. Your input regarding Luise's schooling should be directed to Solvang, according to the guidelines I assume you have. You will continue to be welcome, by arrangement with Solvang, to come to our parties and chat with the teachers here.
Sincerely,
Christian Pedersen

I wrote to the school precisely because the treatment center prevented me from attending school events.

Luise, I want you to know that it made me terribly unhappy to see how you were misunderstood and mistreated. The feeling that you would end up paying for what I did was very painful. The reason I chose not to intervene was to protect you.

I didn't want any part in having you go to more meetings with the authorities where you would again fall flat on your face.

17

DOCUMENTS PILE UP

'But you cannot pluck the stars from heaven...'
'No. But I can put them in the bank.'
'Whatever does that mean?'
'That means that I write the number of my stars on a piece of paper.'
'And then I put this paper in a drawer and lock it with a key.'
'And that is all?'
'That is enough,' said the businessman.

Antoine de Saint-Exupéry, *The Little Prince*

*But where was your caseworker in all this? She documented page
after page, primarily based on the treatment home's many com-
munications. She had supposedly known you for many years. She
had made numerous decisions about your life, but her knowledge came only through contact with other public agencies. The
reality was that she had never actually met you.*

I was occasionally called in to a follow-up conference to discuss
Luise's case.

One such meeting took place in January 1986. I did not know the
purpose of the meeting ahead of time, but sitting there I was asked if I
wanted to be relieved of having Luise home for weekends and holidays.
I didn't understand the question. I was already missing her incredibly
every day, so why would I seek relief from having her home? I remember
it was a very odd but instructive session. It later turned out that I'd been
summoned on the basis of a report from the treatment center.

The letter is full of absolute nonsense. Of course I didn't take Luise
off her medication on weekends, as it says in the letter.

Wouldn't it have been more rational to let me know the letter's contents before the conference, so I would know what the caseworker was talking about?

Too bad we never get the chance now to sit down and talk about why it felt like I wasn't helping you. This is the tragedy.

The funny thing is that I can see for myself how you would have responded to my explanation about what really happened when you were in residential treatment. Flashing your wily but loving smile and with a dismissive wave of your hand, you would have said: 'Oh, Mom! Forget it. Director Nielsen was OK. He was very sweet to Lone and Per. He was only doing what he thought was best.'

Thankfully, you were evicted/discharged from the Solvang treatment center on October 3, 1986.

Prior to this, reports were sent to the Social Services headquarters, our local Social Services office, and Bispebjerg Hospital, among others.

I have subsequently seen the five-page letter sent to our local Social Services, which tells about all the effort the center's teachers had invested in you, only to give up because your own mother constantly resisted the education they provided. That's why they recommended you be sent home.

I didn't resist anything. I was just worried that the drugs would destroy you. My fears would later prove to be justified.

To top it all, the employees claimed in the letter that they had been forced to stop giving you Deprakine because your mother had said you shouldn't take it. You yourself were overjoyed to report that you would soon be off the medication. They told you this at Solvang. I believe your version of the story, because you've always taken your medicine without protest, even when you didn't want it.

The staff actually stopped giving you Deprakine from one day to the next. This was simply irresponsible and dangerous. Medication that affects the brain's receptors should be phased out slowly – otherwise nasty side-effects can result.

You also experienced side-effects from the abrupt discontinuation of your medication. They manifested themselves to you as strange things in your head. You said it was as if things got 'cut off.' That meant you couldn't hold on to a thought, or the words you were reading or writing suddenly disappeared. This made you very scared and very sad. These were the side-effects of the epilepsy drugs you'd been taking for the past few years that you'd now suddenly stopped taking.

Patients (children) with EEG changes, unless the significance of these EEG changes can be determined with certainty, should not be treated with medication, as medication can do more harm than good when it produces side-effects.
Viggo Petersen,
Head of Neurophysiology,
Psychological Laboratory at Dianalund Epilepsy Hospital

Luise, you thankfully got out of the psychiatric treatment home where the staff perceived you as an 'irritation factor.'

But their – to say the least – harsh treatment, administered so callously, certainly didn't boost your self-confidence, and it's also quite possible you emerged with lasting side-effects from the epilepsy medication.

When you came home from Solvang on October 3, 1986, you had actually been drug-free for over a month, something I was initially not aware of.

Realizing that the staff, unilaterally and dangerously, had suddenly stopped your medication, I got really anxious. So again we went to the National Hospital.

As mentioned, the new neurologist wrote in your chart on November 10, 1986, that you were doing much better after coming off Deprakine.

This was written two months after Solvang had informed Social Services, as a pretext for expelling you, that they couldn't take responsibility for you because you refused to take the medication which, in their view, you couldn't do without.

From a treatment point of view, on October 3 we were back where we started when, at only 11 years of age, you checked in for treatment at the National Hospital's neurological department.

All you'd had in the meantime was two and a half years of treatment with an anti-epilepsy drug, which had made you at least 55 lbs heavier – and made you aggressive while you were taking it.

So you were in much worse shape in late 1986 than when you started at the National Hospital in 1983. You were now suffering from serious side-effects, which manifested in your head as strange, incomprehensible and frightening things. You'd become grossly overweight. The weight gain had happened so fast that the skin on your abdomen and thighs had split open. You'd been subjected to both physical and psychological abuse at Copenhagen's best – and only – residential psychiatric treatment center.

By now you'd spent years in the treatment system. Since before 1980, the best conditions for your development had been described in minute detail. These conditions had never been met, partly because you had zigzagged through countless different treatment scenarios. To me it seemed like we started from scratch

every time a new practitioner entered the picture, as if the dif-
ferent treatment centers failed to use each other's observations.
Continuity and consistency of treatment was totally lacking,
which would prove disastrous for you.

The documentation built up. I would hazard a guess that there are many thousands of pages of chart notes about Luise floating around in the system. But what good is all this documentation when no one seems to use it?

Social Services is the place where everything – except hospital charts – is gathered together so that money can be allocated for the various treatment phases. But the caseworkers don't collect things. They have no time for this. They document and catalog the paperwork submitted about the case. As far as I can see, no one has overall responsibility or follows up on whether a mode of treatment– and the money for it – are deployed in a way that's appropriate and beneficial to the party involved.

18

HOPE WANES

I had been conditioned by my own public education.
I was resigned and accepting. There was no choice.
The 'treatment' looked great on paper, in the chart notes.
Then again, it was the caseworkers
and bureaucrats writing it up.

All children long to be loved, appreciated and reassured that they are good at something. You were loved and appreciated by your family and by your friends and my friends. I'm sure you knew this. But like all children, you also needed confirmation of your self-worth from outside this support network. You never got this. Quite the opposite.

At the childcare facility you couldn't conform to the rules of group-based education, so you were referred to a psychologist. This is when Social Services came into the picture for the first time, as they had to allocate money for it. The psychologist found nothing wrong with you, so we were discharged after two visits and advised to change nursery school. This psychological evaluation was never sent to Social Services, as far as I can tell from the records I have gathered.

During all the years they were trying to diagnose you, you repeatedly had to sit and listen to me talking to different specialists about all the things you could NOT do.

Your time at Solvang certainly didn't bolster your sense of actually being good at something.

My friend Anni said often: 'Luise is an amazing girl. She has charisma, determination and intelligence, things that can be of great benefit to her in life.' Anni's opinion unfortunately couldn't make up for all the negative experiences you had.

All those years of 'help' had brought us to the point where we now had to avoid therapists.

I was summoned to a meeting at Social Services in early November 1986. You had been expelled from Solvang, and it was up for debate what should happen now. Medical professionals from the National Hospital also attended on this occasion. In pride of place sat two employees from your former institution, and they had the first word. They started by telling how much you liked your time there, but how difficult it had been to work with me. They said: 'Dorrit didn't want to Luise to take the epilepsy medication because she was afraid that it would make Luise's hair curly.'

You can just imagine how all the participants in the meeting, except my companion, laughed at this deceitful little story. This was real public disparagement. Some time earlier I had mentioned that Luise had experienced all the usual documented side-effects of epilepsy medication – that even her hair was different. This is a rare and, of course, totally inconsequential side-effect. But why did the experts even allow so much discussion about your epilepsy medication? Hadn't they been informed that you weren't taking it anymore? And why did your caseworker say nothing? Several possible treatment centers were suggested but rejected because they were for the mentally retarded.

It wasn't a very reassuring exchange that took place around that table. I was speechless after the humiliating remark about curly hair, and the only thing I would say was that you were doing well and we both wanted you to be at home. This was accepted.

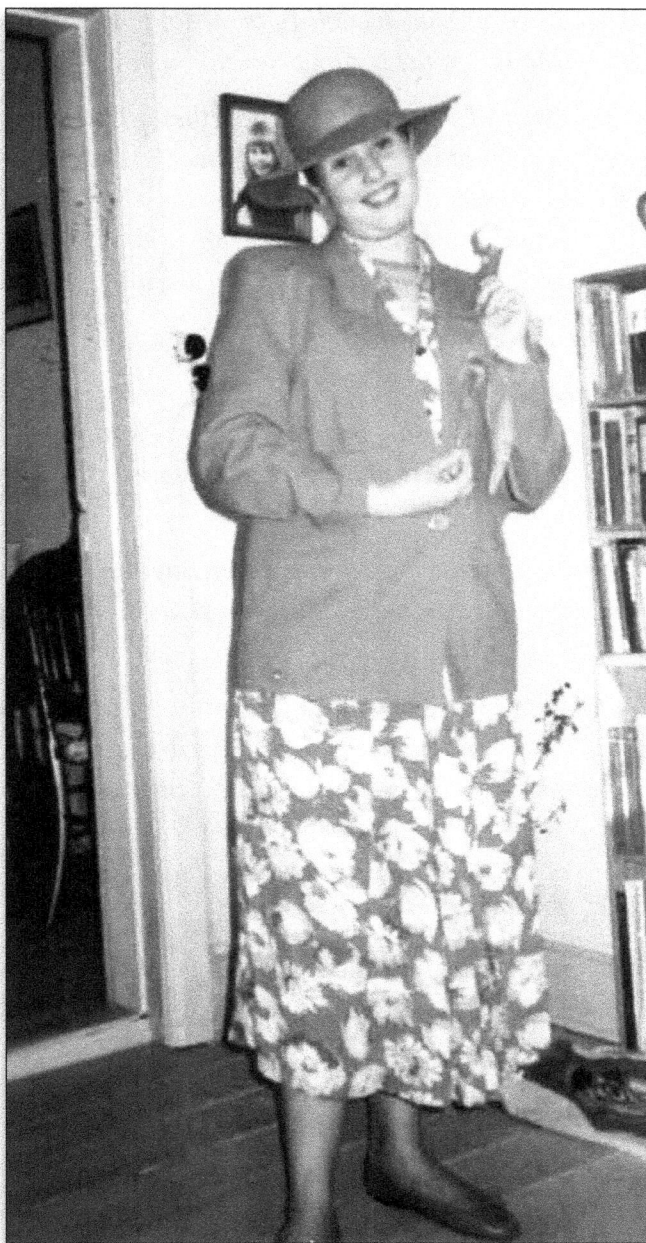

Luise doing her Queen Margrethe impersonation.

You started at the special school. In terms of school experience, you had jumped out of the frying pan into the fire.

The so-called special schools brought together all the pupils who, for one reason or another, couldn't get placed in the regular public schools. This meant that there could be every kind of kid, from very gifted, maladjusted students to severe underperformers, all in the same class. It was quite a disorderly learning environment.

You couldn't concentrate when there was unrest in the class.

You often had headaches and got dizzy. You reported feeling that things got 'cut off' in your brain. When this happened, everything disappeared. For example, the text you were reading would suddenly vanish.

The teachers didn't believe you could learn anything. Their school reports talked very negatively about your skills and your motivation to learn.

The school was not particularly willing to listen to my view that you couldn't concentrate because of disturbances in the classroom, and therefore couldn't benefit from their educational offerings. The school was in no way interested in hearing about the problems you experienced because of 'clutter in my head,' as you called it.

The Institute of Psychology re-entered the picture in 1987 with a new psychological evaluation.

Minutes of the evaluation sent to Social Services – slightly abbreviated:

Conclusion of Psychological Study, June 1987.
Luise can still be described as a delicate girl with easily triggered anxiety, which causes her efforts to become erratic, hesitant and somewhat persistent. She often has trouble getting a grip on a situation, does not feel she has control of it. She often gives up easily and has no confidence she can do anything that is 'good enough'.

Her self-esteem, in other words, is not very high. Based on the psychological study undertaken, I must conclude that Luise still needs a supportive and caring environment that can provide the special considerations her development and functioning require. An essential prerequisite to getting help for Luise is that it takes a form the mother will find acceptable.

Sincerely,

Ole Svendsen

The supportive and caring environment that could meet the special requirements for your development required didn't exist at the special school.

You became ever more discouraged and felt even worse. You were losing faith that you could learn anything at all. I had a feeling that you were about to give up. This feeling unfortunately proved to be correct. On June 6, 1988, you couldn't stand being inside your strange head any more. You took a load of pills.

When I came home from work, I found you lying on the couch. You were watching your favorite film Footloose, *a teen movie with good music. Although peace and harmony filled the air, I could tell that something was terribly wrong. You told me to go visit my friends, so you could enjoy the movie in peace and quiet. I had a distinct feeling I shouldn't leave you alone, so I stayed. It was a wise decision, because a little later you went limp and fell into a deep sleep. I called Peter, a friend in Brumleby. By the time he came you were almost unconscious. We carried you down to a taxi and drove to the National Hospital emergency, where you had your stomach pumped.*

When you woke up, you explained that your suicide attempt happened because you couldn't bear to live with all the strange things going on in your head.

Your chart of June 6, 1988, reports: 'Well-developed puberty-age girl – drowsy, easily awakened. Responds adequately, albeit extremely briefly. Volunteers that her head is not working.'

This showed clearly it was incredibly important for you to get your message across about your 'strange head.' But the neurologist did not take this seriously. She suggested you should go to Bispebjerg Hospital's adolescent psychiatric ward. Our previous experience at this place had been very negative. We feared that if you went there, everything could start all over again, with anti-epileptic medication and the Solvang residential home. We devoted all our energy to ensuring that your two-and-a-half-year nightmare would not be repeated. So we both said no – and for once we were heard.

I again started thinking you must be suffering from absence seizures/hidden epilepsy. You thought so, too. Your perception that things 'got cut off' fit with the description we had of what happens when your mind goes blank due to an epileptic event.

It can be difficult to make the correct diagnosis. The doctor was sure that you suffered from epilepsy. She obviously should have been aware that the medication made you worse, especially when you received such a high dose that almost sent you into spasm.

After two and a half years your medication was stopped from one day the next. Then strange things started to happen inside your head.

Today, 20 years too late, I've learned this was a severe side-effect caused by the anti-epileptic treatment. I didn't know that in 1986.

You had suffered a minor brain injury due to negligent treatment.

I understand that doctors can make medical mistakes. Unfortunately, it's probably unavoidable with their busy work schedule.

On the other hand, I simply cannot understand why they evade responsibility when they've made a mistake. It is immoral.

The doctors should obviously have taken responsibility for the harm you suffered and given you corrective treatment. Today we get very good results when we treat children with minor brain damage – and this was also the case in 1980.

19

Epilepsy hospital

Documentation piles up.
Nobody reads the documents.
The people the documents are about
don't know their contents
and therefore cannot act on them.

We asked that you again be tested for epilepsy. We hoped that an-
other drug might help you get your head straight. Our wish was
granted. You were referred to Filadelfia, the epilepsy hospital.

Luise's evaluation had to focus on why she experienced this horrible sensation in her head, which she described as things getting 'cut
off.' The study got underway at the Filadelfia epilepsy hospital, because
it could be that the strange symptoms were themselves caused by a
kind of epilepsy. Luise was admitted July 14, 1988, and stayed for about
two months.

Her EEG showed extreme fluctuations, but not because of epilepsy,
we learned. We were almost disappointed, for what could it be?

Today I know that the EEG fluctuations could have been due to the
after-effects of the epilepsy medication. But I also know today that people with Asperger's syndrome often have EEG read-outs showing un-
usual fluctuations.

How thrilled you were at the school offerings that came with your
hospital stay. You phoned home and talked excitedly about the
new school subjects you were studying – you had German, Eng-
lish and science, subjects you'd never had at the special school.

Your school reports from Filadelfia were very positive, the exact opposite of reports from the special school.

Excerpts from the school report from Filadelfia, September 14, 1988:
Socially Luise has functioned quite satisfactorily. She has been in a group with four others of her own age. She has had natural, straight-forward dealings with her peers and teachers. Luise is very inter-ested in the world around her and could talk about issues that came up in the classroom, such as pollution, the Iran-Iraq war, etc. Luise has a good attitude and interest in school work. She likes to work independently on her tasks, calling on the teacher only when she needs help or explanation to complete a task. She quickly grasps instruction and can take it to the next step herself. It is important to provide reinforcement that she is a healthy person with good prospects, also career-wise, so that her self-confidence is enhanced.

It was also written that you were good at helping your classmates when they were stuck. Luise, this is only the second official state-ment from your 20 years in treatment in which I can recognize you. The teacher is writing about your strengths. No fault-find-ing, just an empathetic study of you as a person. Luise, you were right when you said you couldn't learn anything when there was too much noise in class. But you were never taken seriously.

The assessment from Filadelfia didn't seem to influence the spe-cial school's earlier perception that your learning abilities and your motivation were lacking.

After Filadelfia your daily life at the special school became in-creasingly onerous for you. You'd seen that you could learn excit-ing new things if you were only taken seriously. You couldn't bear to keep reading the same old books that offered no challenge. Furthermore, the teaching environment had become even more chaotic – if that was possible – and the teachers were perhaps almost giving up. I don't know. They certainly didn't have much sympathy for you.

You were skipping lessons, which got reported to Social Services, and finally it was decided to find another school for you.

We were summoned to yet another meeting. The caseworker had probably not read the report from the epilepsy hospital about how well you could function educationally, indeed when conditions were suitable for you. I only got the papers after your death.

A boarding school by the name of Valdemarsbo was suggested.

Here you could get 'house training,' meaning you could learn to live in your own home.

But you knew how to run a house. You could cook. You knew how to do many things.

You didn't want to go to Valdemarsbo.

You were skeptical at the idea of a 'good place' chosen by the authorities.

This idea brought Solvang to mind.

The psychiatrist at the National Hospital had originally assured us this was a good place.

But you hungered for book knowledge. The stay in Filadelfia had instilled in you the confidence to learn.

We were lucky. There was no room at Valdemarsbo, so this gave us a little time to regroup.

20

A TURNING POINT

*At Tvind they focused on your resources.
There was no fault-finding.
You grew with their teaching.*

The thought of ending up in a place like Valdemarsbo prompted Luise to take matters into her own hands. She found a school in North Jutland, in the Tvind network of experimental schools, which she wanted to go to. I was happy to phone and tell this to her caseworker, and then we just had to deal with the formalities of getting the student grant. It turned out that the Copenhagen municipal authorities would not provide funding for Luise to attend a Tvind school, which put the plan way beyond our means. Luise had finally found a place she felt was right for her, and now I simply couldn't cover the cost without a student grant.

So we took a trip to her prospective new school to talk about the problem. They told us not to worry about it. They could tell that Luise wanted to be there, so they would step in with financial assistance. This meant that I paid what I could and the school paid the rest.

It turned out that Luise made the right choice. Her stay there was a turning point in her life. She received individualized instruction, and she began to learn and learn. She couldn't get enough. She passed the ninth grade oral exam in English, physics and chemistry with good grades. She finished these classes in six months, which was quite an achievement, since she hadn't studied the subjects before. She took computer courses and later took cooking and needlecraft.

Luise spent a couple of years at the Tvind schools in Frederikshavn and then later in Ulfborg. The three years she spent there were good for her.

At Tvind the teachers focused on her resources instead of finding fault. This kind of teaching helped her grow.

Luise made some good friends. She finally took the classes she'd always wanted. She also learned to cook gourmet food and make cool clothes.

Luise was in Norway for an extended period, where she worked as a cook in a mountain hotel. In England she worked for two weeks at a second-hand clothing store. She was in Belgium and Holland and sold things in flea markets.

She was chosen to lead the sales effort at the flea market in Holland because they saw her as an energetic and reliable worker.

Luise sang in the choir and was involved in the Tvind schools' big annual music festival that featured orchestral, choral and solo performances.

This environment was good for Luise, but occasionally she would still go into mental lock-down and say no when asked to do something. She could also get frustrated and shut herself in her room. But the teachers told me, 'Luise is a caring and compassionate girl, and we long since learned that when she says no, and perhaps even goes to her room and locks the door, we just step back. She quickly calms herself, and we've learned from experience that she soon emerges and starts on the task she'd said no to – often with such diligence that she also finishes the work other kids should have done.'

One instance of this was the time when, after a big party, there were so many dishes to wash that nobody could even imagine rising to the task. Luise gave a definite no, so the others followed suit. However, it all ended with Luise doing the dishes. She stayed up half the night and took care of the job by herself. That was just the way Luise was, and they accepted it. The other students were quick to acknowledge Luise's extraordinary effort. She was well liked, and her classmates could accept her special way of being, because she showed empathy for anyone having a hard time.

I remember one spring you showed up at home on an unscheduled visit. You told me you were never going back to school. Apparently you'd had a falling-out with your roommates. You were one of four girls living in a house. No more, you said. But after two days you were already missing them, so you phoned and asked if you could come back. It was OK with them, and you were even lucky enough to find one of the Tvind teachers in Copenhagen you could drive back with. You were welcomed with open arms by your roommates and teachers. None of the usual getting into trouble and being told how serious it was that you'd run away.

Another time you suddenly appeared on the doorstep of my friend Elsebeth, in the middle of nowhere. How on earth had you found your way there? She lived in a small village a few miles from the nearest town, with no public transport. We had only visited Elsebeth once, when we were picked up miles away. But you had an uncanny ability to find your way around the entire country. I have no idea how you did it. Anyway, Elsebeth gave you a cup of tea and you sat and chatted before driving back to the school in Frederikshavn.

I visited you often at the schools in Frederikshavn and Ulfborg. It was always a heartening experience to see all your activities and the enthusiasm you all brought to them. The most fun were your annual day-long musical events, held in Jutland one year and on Zealand (the main island) the next.

In 1991 the event was on Zealand at St. Annæ High School. Your father, uncle Mogens and I were all agreed this would be an experience we'd never forget, listening to great music for 12 hours straight. You Tvind students were in charge of the cooking and serving and the entertainment.

St. Annæ school auditorium and concert hall, which seats approx. 1,000 people, was packed. Arriving around 10 am, we found coffee and homemade cakes waiting for us.

After coffee we went into the great hall and were regaled with wonderful classical music until noon, when we filed out to the beautiful table settings, where we sat and delighted at an exquisite three-course menu that even Copenhagen's Hotel d'Angleterre couldn't improve on.

All you students bustled around us, waiting on us and serving us with maximum professionalism, all dressed in your black pants and white shirts.

Plates were promptly removed after the first course, making room for our next course, and then on to dessert, which you had helped to make. It was heavenly.

Actually, we were stuffed after the main course. But who could resist a dessert that was a beautifully colorful work of art made of homemade ice cream on an almond base, sprinkled with all the multicolored fresh berries that were in season. The homemade mango sauce was dotted with small sprigs of mint forming a crescent. Across from it were doodles in milk chocolate.

You were very busy. Your team had to clear the tables and get ready for the next round of diners, while we sat comfortably and listened to music.

You only had time to talk to us briefly while we had our afternoon coffee. Otherwise you were on your toes the whole time.

The highlight of the festival was the choral work that ends the second act of Gluck's opera, Orpheus and Eurydice. On stage stood at least 200 students from the whole Tvind school network, singing the heroes and heroines choral piece.

You certainly were heroes and heroines.

The whole hall was exhilarated. It was indescribably beautiful.

We wanted an encore, but you felt that we should be satisfied.

We'd been listening to music for 12 hours, interrupted only by the finest food and the best service you can imagine.

By 10 pm you looked pretty tired. Hell, you and your team had been going strong since 5 am, when you started packing the food and table settings to bring to St. Annæ High School. That was at the Roskilde afterschool, where the dessert team had its base.

Now you had to clean up. Tableware, leftover food and anything else had to be cleared before midnight. Then you had to wash all the dishes in Roskilde before you could relax.

Luise, I've always admired the energy that you could sometimes bring to the day. You were results-oriented and could put in a major effort when you saw it had purpose. There was a rationale to sewing a waiter's outfit – it would actually be used. The serving uniforms you all wore when waiting on us at the music festival were the clothes you'd help make in your sewing class.

There was also a point to taking cooking courses, as the food you learned to cook was what you ate in your cafeteria every day. Your exquisite culinary achievements the rest of us could enjoy at events like your big music festivals.

Things went well for you at Tvind. You were respected as the person you were. You regained some of your self-confidence. But would your time there have turned out so beneficial if you'd been gulping down anti-epileptic drugs? I don't think so.

21

'HELP' FROM SOCIAL SERVICES

*To have any chance of leading
a person to a particular place,
one must first and foremost
be sure to meet him where he is
and begin there.*

Søren Kierkegaard

Luise came home from Tvind. She was 19 and stood on the threshold of adulthood.

She had come of age and so had to talk alone with her caseworker about her future and her personal economy.

I was very nervous about how her first interview would go.

From what I could see, Luise had the odds stacked against her. Social Services' longstanding knowledge of her came solely through her file. They had never met her. The thick manila folder bulged with papers from experts that mostly represented Luise as a person with serious psychiatric problems who appeared to have benefited significantly from their medication and environmental therapy.

Social Services most likely does not see hospital medical records. But then there were those letters from the child psychiatry ward, applying for a place at a treatment center for Luise on the grounds that she was very difficult to handle 24 hours a day. There were the letters that Bispebjerg Hospital's youth psychiatry department wrote to Social Services regarding Luise's leaving Solvang. The institution was under Bispebjerg's authority. Among other things, the discharge letter reported that

Luise's development had advanced significantly with the anti-epileptic medication and her stay at Solvang, but unfortunately the mother had obstructed and ruined their good work.

Finally, there were the numerous reports from treatment centers saying the same thing. However, Social Services was not aware of the chart notes from the Neurology Department from 1987, when it appeared Luise had considerably improved after stopping by the anti-epileptic treatment. Nor had they seen the discharge letter of September 15, 1988, after Luise's long stay at Filadelfia, which said: 'The patient has been medication-free while hospitalized. She has enjoyed her stay. She has made good contact with her peers, but she lacks a sense of situation. The patient does not have a strong personality, and it is clear from her demeanor that she has been over-treated. This could have contributed to her perception that she is sick and cannot cope. She is slowly abandoning this self-image, and she must be encouraged to feel she is in good health and has good opportunities, also career-wise, to strengthen her self-confidence.'

I was simply afraid that the many negative expert opinions would make the caseworker propose yet another hospitalization, if the first solo meeting went off track. This course of action had been suggested occasionally.

And I knew that hospitalization could happen with the stroke of a pen, because Luise had been admitted previously.

During all these years I'd been scared that Luise might end up in the mental health system on anti-psychotic drugs. At a conference with the psychologist at the National Hospital in March of 1988 – after Luise had tried to commit suicide and admission to Bispebjerg was suggested – I realize I gave the impression that my biggest fear was that Luise would be diagnosed with schizophrenia if she was hospitalized. I knew she didn't have this condition.

Tony Attwood, a clinician specializing in the diagnosis and treatment of Asperger's syndrome, has written about how easily some of the clinical signs of this condition might confuse psychiatrists, who mistakenly arrive at a diagnosis of schizophrenia. It is easy to see how a false diagnostic trail is created. Unfortunately, as he writes, it is likely that a sizeable proportion of those diagnosed with drug resistance (i.e. the medication does not work as intended) or atypical chronic mental illness are eventually found to have Asperger's syndrome.

Luise, I could see that, despite your many resources developed through several troubled years, you reacted guardedly and uncertainly when you realized the conference was about how you were feeling and how you were managing things. You usually went into your mental lockdown and would refuse to talk about this. I understand that your reaction was caused by the fact that too often you had felt manipulated into 'admitting' that you were to blame for things that were not your fault. For example, there was the matter of your bruised arm at Solvang, where you were accused of improperly reporting a staff member for abuse and ended up 'confessing' the transgression in front of city officials. You knew you had been tricked but were unable to defend yourself in a convincing manner.

So it was no wonder that you reacted guardedly and uncertainly when people wanted to talk about your future.

Children with Asperger's syndrome are often very honest and usually are incapable of cheating and lying, but their honesty makes them vulnerable. They hide nothing from others, and in their naivety often allow themselves to be manipulated by adults and the more sophisticated children.
Ole Sylvester Jorgensen, psychiatrist

How often I'd seen that look in your eyes when, for one reason or another, you felt misunderstood. Your expression would turn strangely perplexed, gloomy and hesitant, as if you were wondering, 'What did I do wrong?' You usually blamed yourself if a conversation went off track. But I also knew that you sometimes got so frustrated that you responded by getting mad or stonewalling the person you had miscommunicated with. I was afraid you would feel pressured and respond inappropriately to your caseworker at the meeting. If that were to happen, I was afraid the Center's psychiatrist might suggest hospitalization at the adolescent psychiatry unit, and the whole medication thing would start over again.

So I wanted to give the caseworker the opportunity to get to know you as the lovely and resourceful person you were. I wanted to tell him that you had learning potential in spite of poor school reports. You were inquisitive and often sat at home looking things up in encyclopedias and dictionaries. And it was important that you get support so you could take advantage of the strengths mentioned in reports from the Institute of Psychology. Reports from Filadelfia had also pointed out that you had wide-ranging knowledge.

I simply wanted you to get off to a good start. And, in all honesty, I was afraid that this crucial first session would go badly. I also knew you were nervous about having to go to the interview because of your previous degrading experiences with officialdom.

I wanted to set up a preliminary meeting, hopefully to pave the way for you to have a successful first session.

Your caseworker didn't think it was a good idea for us to meet first. You were now an adult, and I had to let go. No doubt he said this to protect you, and because he thought he had the necessary information on you in the file.

I discussed my concerns about your future with our family doctor. She suggested you should have a psychiatric evaluation, so you could get the 'paperwork' updated about what you were good at and what you needed help with. She told us that if we made the application ourselves, your 'case' would look better because we had taken the initiative. We were both happy with the proposal.

It might sound paradoxical that once again we were daring to take on the psychiatric care system. But we did it precisely to avoid what for us would be the worst outcome imaginable – that you would be hospitalized with Social Services' blessing, meaning you most likely would be considered a psychiatric patient and duly medicated. So we chose the lesser of two evils by applying for the evaluation ourselves.

But you can't just walk up to the reception desk in the psychiatry department and ask for a psychiatric evaluation. You have to be referred by a doctor and have a legitimate reason for the referral – though the situation is obviously different if you have an acute mental condition.

Coincidentally, there had been a minor episode while we were at our summerhouse in Kulhuse two weeks after you got home from Tvind. You believed that three of your good school friends from Tvind were coming to visit us – John, Michael and Jonathan from Zambia. They had visited us six months earlier in Copenhagen. But we had made no arrangements with your three friends to visit us this time. So it was a delusion, to use the psychiatric terminology. It meant that you mistakenly thought something was about to happen.

I'm sure most people have had delusions in one form or another. We've all been in situations where we thought a friend had purposely done something to annoy or deceive us. Or we might have mistakenly heard someone promise us something we really wanted. In either case we might be wrong and simply think of it as paranoia or wishful thinking. But if you're a psychiatric patient, it's considered delusional.

In the circumstances, we chose to call your expectation of friends visiting a delusion, because it might serve as a starting point to getting referred for psychiatric evaluation. So on July 18, 1992, I called our family doctor from the summer house. She believed that the delusions you'd experienced provided a good enough reason to get you admitted for the evaluation. This proved correct. That evening we showed up with our referral at the reception desk at the National Hospital's psychiatry department.

At midnight it was our turn, and – oblivious of what it might lead to – you told the visiting psychiatrist about your notion that school friends from Tvind were coming to visit us. You very convincingly explained that you didn't want medication, because you couldn't tolerate it. You talked about your bad experiences with anti-epileptic medication, how it had made you aggressive and made your brain stop working. You'd become very fat from this drug. I confirmed your explanation.

For us it was crucial that your chart indicate no psychotropic drugs were to be administered during your hospital stay and that you were there just for observation.

The psychiatrist could hear that you had delusions. She also felt that they didn't cause you distress and that you could actually correct yourself and say you knew your friends weren't really coming. But you did experience it, perhaps because you were missing them. The psychiatrist also said it was not uncommon to see people have delusions during periods of stress. This certainly fit your situation. You'd just been on a school trip to Amsterdam. There you'd had responsibility for a large flea market, which undoubtedly had been a demanding task for you.

We didn't leave the room before hearing the visiting physician record all our information plus her observations in the dictation machine for later transcription to your chart.

We were very heartened by the meeting, and you were optimistic about being admitted for evaluation. I walked home in the lovely warm July night – you could even say I danced all the way home. I was excited at the prospect that things had taken a turn for the better for you.

I sat in my kitchen with a cup of tea and let ideas fly around in my head. I could now see you finishing your education, with a little back-up for your special needs. You had several options open to you. It might be something to do with animals. You liked being with animals and were good with them, so why couldn't you aim for a career where you had daily contact with animals? You might also consider an academic education. My imagination ran away with me.

I had to repeatedly tell myself, 'Relax, Dorrit. It's Luise's life, not yours.' But my dreams knew no bounds that lovely July night in 1992.

With the wisdom of hindsight I now realize it might have been better for Luise to meet her caseworker, even with the odds stacked against her, and taken our chances there.

But as Danish citizens we're brought up to believe that you can always safely turn to the health care system and get qualified help. Naturally, we had trust in the system – with fatal consequences.

22

NEW LABEL: 'SCHIZOPHRENIC'

*'Within the diagnostic culture all behavior can in principle
be interpreted as symptoms of the presumed illness.
A patient's utterances, assertions and emotional expression
are seen as signs of inner mental processes
that in turn are caused by the illness.'*

Chief Physician Finn Jørgensen

*On the afternoon of July 19, the day after our meeting to discuss
your evaluation, your godmother Bodil and I visited you in the
psychiatric ward at the National Hospital.*

*We were greeted by a shocking sight. We found you lying on the
floor in your own urine. You were angry and ashamed that we
should see you in this humiliating condition. You said that staff
wouldn't help you get to the toilet and you fell when you tried to
get out of bed by yourself.*

*My first reaction was that this couldn't possibly be true. But it cer-
tainly was true, as I learned when I asked the nurse in charge of you.
She said simply: 'Luise can get up OK. She's just horsing around to
get attention. We've tried to help her several times, but she keeps letting herself fall.' The hint was that this happened on purpose.*

*Bodil and I tried to help you up into bed, but your legs had gone
limp. You actually couldn't stand on them. I didn't understand
what had happened. Why the sudden change?*

*I got really scared when you said you'd been given strong medica-
tion, and that was why you couldn't stand on your own two feet.*

I approached the hospital staff and asked what kind of medicine they'd given you. They wouldn't tell me. I thought, 'This simply can't be right.' You had presented yourself for psychiatric evaluation the previous night. You weren't distressed or agitated, and we were promised you wouldn't get any drugs. And here I find you the next day so heavily medicated.

I was convinced there had been a mistake. It was just a matter of getting hold of the doctor you'd consulted the previous night, so the 'mistake' could be rectified. Fortunately, she was on the ward that day, so the misunderstanding could easily be dealt with, I thought. But I soon learned better, when the doctor wouldn't talk to me. She waved me off with the excuse that she didn't have the time.

You were understandably angry and desperate, telling me: 'It's you who got me in here. You need to get me out of here and it has to be right now!' Your speech was muffled and slow, a clear sign of heavy medication.

I was terribly shocked to see you in this state, and the only solution I could see was to try to talk with the doctor the following day. I promised you that what I saw as a mistake would be corrected.

You reluctantly went along with this.

The next day the doctor was not on the ward, and my promise that you would be drug-free had to be pushed forward to the following day.

I had no idea that all the data the visiting psychiatrist had dictated into the recording machine was never written into your chart. So no one knew you were in for observation without medication.

I just don't understand how the psychiatrists on the ward where you were admitted hadn't wondered why a patient was suddenly dumped on them without any paperwork.

In fact, this meant they didn't know why you were admitted, or whether you'd previously been hospitalized, or whether you'd ever been on psychotropic medication before. For that matter, they'd no idea whether you suffered from a physical illness that might indicate you couldn't tolerate such drugs. And there was a lot of other crucial data the doctors didn't have.

It didn't seem to make any difference to them that they lacked important information that should have formed the basis for any treatment or observation. I could see this when I finally got your chart notes in January 2001. Here it almost seems like they thought you were from another psychiatric ward.

For example, the July 19 chart note from a few hours after your admission states: 'Continued increase in Cisordinol tablet to 10 mg, twice daily, with possible higher dose later.' This had to refer to an ongoing treatment with Cisordinol. But you weren't getting any such treatment. You'd never taken this kind of drug. And you'd stopped taking anti-epileptic medication four years earlier.

So without any prior examination you got a large dose of antipsychotic medication. This was tantamount to a doctor giving someone a large dose of antihypertensive medication without first having checked the patient's blood pressure!

Luise, nothing indicated that you needed antipsychotics. You were not distressed. You were not a danger to yourself or others, but calm and quiet. You were not forced to go to the hospital, you had gone voluntarily.

Mental illnesses cannot be measured using equipment or tests. A psychiatrist makes a diagnosis based on clinical evaluation, which in turn means that the patient's condition and its severity are assessed solely by the psychiatrist based on patient interviews.

Below are all the things the psychiatrist on the ward committed to paper in your chart after his first conversation with you a few hours after you were admitted. He makes the most far-fetched observations.

He must have asked questions whose intent you may not have completely understood, and mostly requiring a simple YES or NO answer.

I really don't know. I can only say that you had been very straightforward the night before and didn't have any of the undermentioned attributes, except a mild form of delusion.

Attributes noted in chart dated July 19 1992:
   Paranoid delusions
   Auditory hallucinations
   Mind controlled by outside forces
   People gossip about you
   When you look in the mirror, you see a witch instead of yourself
   Slightly diminished intellectually capacity
   Emotional communication impaired
   Appears anxious and distressed
   Self-referring conceptualization
   Thought disorder
   Depersonalization
   Derealization
   Talks about suicide because of extreme anxiety

You couldn't possibly have expressed or shown signs of these 13 symptoms. Indeed, I don't think we could find any person showing all these symptoms at one time.

The psychiatrist's questioning technique must have been guided by his preconceived expectations, which led to symptom descriptions verging on the absurd.

Finn Jørgensen's statement from 1970 comes very close: 'Within the diagnostic culture all behavior can in principle be interpreted as symptoms of the presumed illness.'

But as soon as the psychiatrist had enshrined these symptoms in your chart, they seemed to be automatically transformed into gospel truth. And this would form the basis for your continuing treatment.

What on earth was happening? I simply didn't get it. My reluctance to be suspicious must be viewed in light of my confidence that clear-headed and well thought-out treatment was underway, albeit with a misunderstanding that had to be corrected. I had no knowledge of the chart notes recording the 13 severe schizophrenic symptoms, which were first written down just after you were admitted.

From that first evening on I never managed to get hold of the doctor.

When I came to visit you on the fifth day, I learned you'd been moved to St. Hans Hospital. I probably just nodded and asked for the address, and then made my way there to visit you.

Today I realize how enraged I was to see you in that state. Had I been able to think clearly, I might have sensed something was seriously amiss. This couldn't be normal procedure. A person admitted for a 14-day psychiatric evaluation obviously should not be transferred to another hospital in the middle of the process. But my state of shock made it impossible for me to get a grip on the situation, Luise.

It felt as if I was constantly running around after things I couldn't identify. I found myself in a constant state of stress as I watched what was happening to my sweet girl.

At St. Hans they knew nothing of the 'psychiatric evaluation without any medication.'

I told the psychiatrist in your ward that I was sure you couldn't tolerate such high doses of medication. The response was simply that you were being properly medicated. Our exchange took place in a friendly tone, but the underlying implication was that

I shouldn't meddle in their treatment.

Visiting you the next day, I could see things were about to go terribly wrong, and it was getting worse by the day. You were starting to get very strange. You moved hesitantly and you'd become very distant. You'd started walking with short shuffling steps, arms outstretched like a sleepwalker. You fell all the time and couldn't even get up by yourself. I was now in a state of panic, which obviously irritated the staff. For five days I'd been telling the psychiatrist you obviously couldn't tolerate the drug, but in vain. When I came to visit you on the sixth day, they'd taken you to the emergency ward at Roskilde Hospital. There I found you all hooked up with tubes and needles, and you were blue and yellow all over your body. You'd had a severe reaction to the medication – you were suffering from neuroleptic malignant syndrome (NMS), a drug poisoning from the antipsychotic medication. I now know that this is a serious condition that often ends in death.

Ten days after being hospitalized for a brief psychiatric evaluation you ended up getting drug poisoning. And I hadn't been able to do anything about it.

23

NATIONAL HOSPITAL

Had your mind left this world forever?
I was desperate, I froze up inside,
walked around in a strange fog.

*I was at my wits' end. You were totally changed after this vio-
lent medical reaction. Physically you were very weak, walked in-
decisively and fell often. You were in another world where you
couldn't be reached. Your eyes were lifeless, and your facial fea-
tures rigid. You couldn't talk. Everything within reach you stuffed
in your mouth. It could be cigarette butts, apple cores, bottle tops.
You were like a big baby. When you had to go to the toilet, you
paraded through the entire ward with your pants around your
ankles, yelling at the staff: 'I have to pee! Come and help me!'*

*At the same time you'd become very aggressive, and your anger
was directed especially at me. Understandably, for I had gone
along with getting you hospitalized. In any case, they would have
taken drastic 'punitive measures' if your aggression had been directed towards the hospital staff.*

*I was afraid that you, my beloved Luise, had mentally left this
world forever. I was desperate, I froze up inside, walked around in
a strange fog. I never thought of speaking out, asking questions or
holding anyone responsible for this instance of serious malpractice.*

*You were watched around the clock by medical students. I spoke
with one of the students who took care of you. He thought you
were severely mentally retarded. He was surprised to hear that
barely a month earlier you'd been in Amsterdam, managing sales*

at a flea market. He was outraged that the staff hadn't told him what had happened to you, because he got the impression you were profoundly debilitated and had treated you accordingly.

I first found out in 2001, when I got access to your medical records, that the initial consultation on July 18, 1992, the night you were hospitalized, was never entered into your chart. I could also now see that the information we gave about your probably not being able to tolerate antipsychotics had been lifted to another meeting on August 4 between me and the examining psychiatrist. That meeting never took place. I never got to talk to the examining psychiatrist, despite my persistent attempts. This is simply a falsification of the record. There must have been a reason. I cannot see any other reason than that they were aware they had made a mistake by giving you large doses of medication, despite our warnings that you couldn't tolerate it. They sought to cover up this mistake by pretending that we shared this information with them after the drug poisoning.

After two days at Roskilde County Hospital Luise returned to the National Hospital ward where the whole debacle began.

If you read about neuroleptic malignant syndrome in the medical journals, you'll see that it says: 'In cases of NMS, antipsychotics should be discontinued immediately and the patient transferred without delay to intensive care for treatment of these symptoms.' Then the statement: 'In some cases it ends with the irreversible neurological defects.' Luise never got into intensive care. No one took account of her very serious condition. No one acted as if there was a possibility of irreversible neurological defects.

Within a few days they again started giving you anti-psychotic medication. It was far too soon, considering how shattered you were. You had not nearly recovered from the after-effects of the drug poisoning. You were incontinent, you had a fever and your blood pressure was far too high. Blood tests showed elevated levels of creatinine phosphokinase. This level had been up to 15,780, now supposedly falling but still not down to normal, which is between 40 and 80. You still went around like a sleepwalker. It says in your chart from August 3, 1992: 'Needs help with all practical things. Has odd eating habits, yesterday ate paper, cigarette butts and whatever else lay around.'

Your care team must have 'forgotten' that you'd been seriously poisoned five days earlier and this was the reason for your strange behavior. Instead, they saw you as insane, and their only response to this was more medicine.

You refused to take the pills, as they wrote in your chart: 'The patient refuses to take medication because she states she has received so much medication that she has got sick from it, which is why she no longer wants it.' This chart note is from August 17, 1992, less than a month after you were hospitalized. What you said was true. Fourteen days earlier you had almost died from the drug. The psychiatrist chose to construe as psychotic drivel your claim that you got sick from the medicine.

On August 20: 'It was decided today to conduct mandated treatment with an injection of Roxiam. The patient was informed of complaint procedures, but the patient has expressed no desire to appeal to the Patient Complaints Commission.'

Then for an extended period (20 days) you were subjected to mandated daily medication.

Luise, while still suffering the after-effects from the poisoning how could you be in a fit state to file a patient complaint? Didn't it almost feel like they were making fun of you with such an offer?

The August 20 chart also states: 'Dominant in the patient is a very low level of cognition, while her reaction patterns show her to be severely regressed and hysterical.'

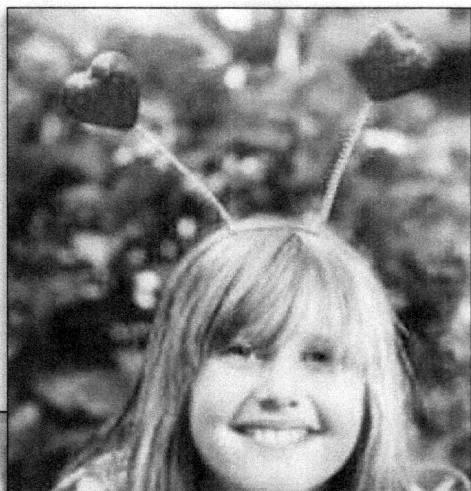

*Luise in Hyde Park, London; with
Johanna in Brumleby.*

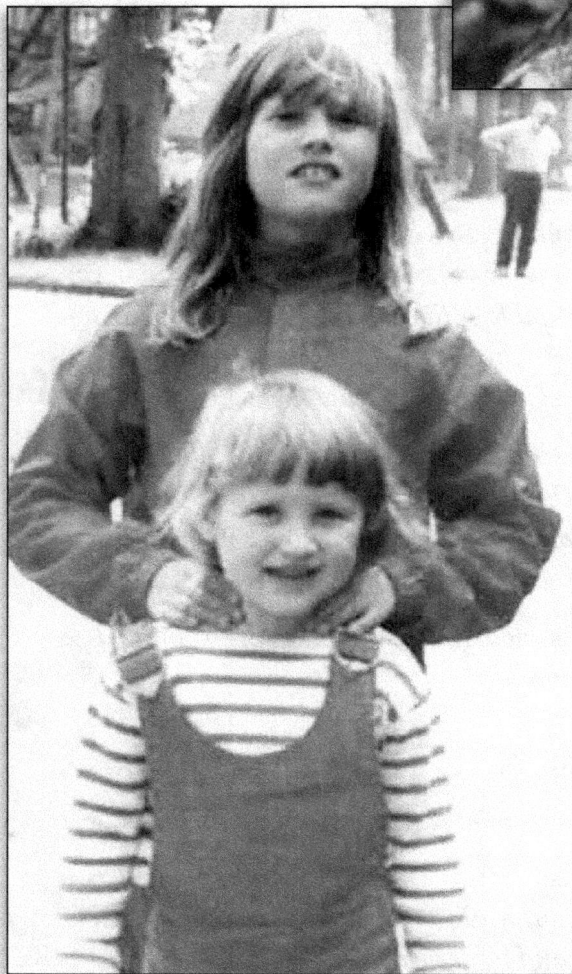

In one month, according to records, your intellectual level had now changed from 'a slight cognitive impairment' to 'a very low level of intelligence.'

Chart note from July 19, one month earlier: 'One gets the impression of a slight cognitive impairment.' Such a rapid cognitive collapse is unthinkable. Unless it's caused by a severe acute brain illness. If you read up on the symptoms of encephalitis, for example, you'll find a pattern that fits your reaction – indeed, a pattern of serious and rare symptoms requiring urgent action.

Your very frightening reaction was obviously caused by the drug poisoning, but I was never informed of this.

I was invited to meet with the chief psychiatrist and a couple of senior doctors after you'd developed neuroleptic malignant syndrome. They tried to calm me down and smooth things over. Among other things, the doctors told me that your poor condition was transitory and most likely harder on me than on you. They justified it by saying that you would forget what had happened. I didn't understand what they meant by forgetting what had happened. Their explanation was that you wouldn't be able to remember how you'd become progressively worse until you finally ended up in a coma. You would forget you'd been just like a baby and ate cigarette butts and the like. And the fact that you'd threatened me with all sorts of misfortunes would also be eradicated from your mind.

Here, at least, was some compensation, because I could only wish that these terrible experiences be purged from your consciousness.

But it turned out that you remembered every detail from before, during and after the drug poisoning. You could describe the horrifying sensation of gradually losing control of yourself, as you finally slid into a coma. Unfortunately, you also remembered all the strange things you said and did in your toxic state.

You were embarrassed by your strange behavior, which included eating cigarette butts, and by your extremely bizarre conduct in general (as they put it in your chart). I learned all this after you started to feel more like yourself. You rattled on about your friends who had visited you while you were weird and said you didn't want them to visit you again. You were so ashamed that they'd seen you in that condition and you didn't think you could look them in the eye again.

So you were certainly not oblivious of what had happened.

There were simply so many frightful things involved in Luise's treatment that I had to 'archive' them deep in my subconscious just so I could get through the day. I probably was a very trusting and compliant mother. I never really had any choice, because everything was so overwhelmingly awful.

Chart note, August 21, 1992: 'The mother is obviously worried that the patient requires mandated treatment, but declares she has never seen the patient in this state. The mother supports the department's belief that it is necessary to administer mandated treatment to ensure that the condition does not become chronic.'

Well of course I gave my approval for the mandated treatment. The alternative, according to the psychiatrist, was that your terrible condition would be permanent! You simply weren't in this world. So I would go along with anything to get you back.

I didn't know any better, and I was sick with sorrow and despair at seeing you suffer. Had I known what I know today, I would certainly have said no.

August 24, 1992, the psychiatrist noted: 'I had a conversation today with the mother, who cannot have contact with the patient, as the patient is violent and paranoid towards her. The mother is obviously rather distraught at the situation but totally concurs with our treatment plan. I explain that if the condition has not changed in the next few days, it may be necessary to implement ECT therapy, which the mother also accepts.'

Luise, I was scared witless at the thought of your getting electro-shock treatment. I was frightened to death. I can't even imagine what you were going through.

It slowly dawned on me that the doctors intended to act as if you never had neuroleptic malignant syndrome. I could hear this in my conferences with them. Today I see it in the chart notes. They didn't want to try and initiate treatment to counteract the NMS. Rather, they had 'forgotten' that you had been poisoned. Now they chose to interpret your very poor condition as a sign of a rapidly progressing deterioration in your mental state rather than as a result of the drug poisoning.

Luise, you said on August 17 that you didn't want the medicine, because you'd had so much medication it had made you ill. You were right.

I am left with the very depressing thought that all Luise's pain could have been avoided if the doctors had simply been willing take responsibility for their mistakes.

First, Luise gets drug poisoning because they don't take seriously our warnings that she can't tolerate anti-psychotic medication. It's now clear to me that they are aware from the start that there has been a mistake, which should be concealed at all costs. This is achieved by a chart entry about a conference that never took place. Once the damage is done, they do nothing to deal with it. Luise is not detoxified in the intensive care unit, as required by regulations, and in the end they do nothing to treat the irreversible neurological damage she has obviously suffered.

The August 20 chart note saying that her dominant trait was a very low level of cognition may well have been a sign of this. It makes shivers run down my spine to think that they'd even contemplated giving Luise electroshock treatment. How could they possibly visit such treatment on a person whose brain is already destroyed by drug poisoning? I now have to say that the care providers had a sadly diminished sense of responsibility. Errors are concealed behind by fake chart notes. The cause of the misery is forgotten. Now they say Luise's condition was caused by a progression of the disease, and that can only be treated with more medication.

24

Coercion doesn't work

*Today the patient offers no physical resistance
but is anxious about being medicated and holds hands,
and afterwards she is somewhat tearful.*

Reading Luise's 600-page chart is a wretched experience. It presents an impersonal diagnosis, with signs of coercion, both direct and indirect, permeating the stack of chart notes.

She is repeatedly told that she's very ill, and if she doesn't take the proposed medication she will get even sicker. Who would dare oppose an increased dosage? Luise certainly didn't dare. She opposed the large doses of medication at first, but this always resulted in mandated treatment, so she eventually stopped resisting.

On October 29, 1992 she was again transferred to St. Hans Hospital. Right away she said no to drugs on the grounds that they were making her ill. Shortly afterwards the mandated medication began – administered by syringe – along with periodic use of belt restraints.

After 12 days she was broken – November 11, 1992: 'Today the patient offers no physical resistance but is anxious about being medicated and holds hands, and afterwards she is somewhat tearful.'

I visited Luise three times a week.

Staff at the unit where she was fastened in restraints and forcibly medicated told me that I should always phone before visiting.

*As they put it, 'It's best for Luise that she's prepared for a visit.'
You were never in restraints when I visited you, Luise. You never told me you were strapped down a great deal of the time.*

Why was that?

Did you really believe I knew what was going on and just did nothing to help you?

Or did you simply think it was too painful to talk about? Or was it because you didn't want to upset me?

I'll never know.

Luise, I got chills when I read the 2001 chart note indicating you were anxious and tearful at the abusive treatment. The wording suggested to me that for the psychiatrists it was a matter of 'wearing down a victim.' In this case it was through coercion. There was no sign that the psychiatrist felt he should talk to you, despite your distress and tears.

Luise had been medicated erroneously with antipsychotics from day one. After ten days she was at death's door from this treatment. Her brain had undoubtedly been seriously damaged by the drug poisoning. The obvious response should surely have been rehabilitation, as would be the norm in other medical specialties when treating patients in this state. Instead, Luise was injected with large doses of medication – the worst thing imaginable.

The doctors had doubts about her diagnosis for the first two years. The psychiatrist told me in a conference, 'Luise can't be schizophrenic because she hasn't followed normal schizophrenic development.'

I said I was sure Luise's problems had nothing to do with schizophrenia. But then I was stuck when they asked me: 'So what do you think is wrong with Luise?' I didn't know, but I'd hoped the care providers could figure that out. I could tell them that Luise had been a wonderful girl ever since she was born but was a bit 'different' and that I dearly wished she could get a diagnosis that fit her so she could be helped to get on with her life with the right education. I also pointed out that the medical treatment she'd so far received had made her much worse. This conversation gave me a little hope. A psychiatrist was asking questions and listening.

The conference changed a few things. Dosage was cut in half and Luise got somewhat better.

At St. Hans Hospital Luise was diagnosed with paranoid psychosis. Many people may have episodes of paranoid psychosis, and the prognosis is good for this condition.

In early February, Luise was released for a week to come home and help with the move into her new apartment in Brumleby.

On February 17, 1993, I had a conversation with a psychiatrist and reported that the move went well. I also told him that Luise's worst side-effects had moderated. We arranged for her to come home to the apartment and stay for short periods.

There were already plans for Luise's transition around New Year, and full discharge was expected in the summer. In the spring we would have a discussion about the kind of support she needed.

The February 18 treatment plan states, 'Discharged gradually to own home. Can stay at home in own apartment for periods and then return. We expect final discharge in early June.'

Luise couldn't wait to get home and sometimes came home without arranging it with the hospital. She had always been impulsive.

On April 3 Luise made the trip home without arranging it first. We went back together. We met a new psychiatrist, who noted: 'The patient seems distressed when approached, seems locked inside herself, keeps her mouth in a simulated pucker, possibly experiences auditory hallucinations, is oriented in time and place, seems detached.'

Now Luise was suddenly subject to mandatory confinement, both as a safety measure and a treatment necessity. The drug dose increased dramatically and was administered under duress, and she was strapped down.

This forced treatment continued for many days.

This just couldn't be right. A few days before Luise was about to be discharged, she meets a new psychiatrist who shouts fire. Everything changes. I don't know the circumstances, but perhaps Luise got angry, or maybe she was simply punished for going home early. Outside the walls we can permit ourselves to be angry and go wherever we wish. If you're inside the walls and don't obey, then you're dangerous and get mandatory medication while you're strapped down in bed.

The mandatory medication and restraints continued until April 26. During this period Luise was also denied freedom of movement. This meant she had no fresh air for 22 days.

After the mandatory treatment was finished, Luise was given leave to take a half-hour outside.

Luise headed for home and would not return.

The chart note for May 4, 1993, states: 'Since the patient is discharged, mandatory treatment is discontinued.'

25

FREE FROM HALLUCINATION

*Your beautiful mind
and your good judgment
protected you.*

Many years ago I told your psychologist, Ole Svendsen, that I was nervous that your open mind and trust in strangers might allow some people to take advantage of you and hurt you.

Ole Svendsen said I had to trust that your good judgment and your beautiful mind would protect you.

He was right.

You had always managed well, even in the toughest situations.

After the 22 days of forced treatment you'd taken the matter into your own hands. On April 27, 1993, you left for your apartment in Brumleby. There was no way you would ever go back for forced drugging or drug poisoning, as you put it. I was terribly scared by the thought that you'd stopped taking the anti-psychotic medication from one day to the next, having learned how dangerous this could be. Do you remember how I tried everything to persuade you to return to the hospital? But you weren't going to change your mind. You'd had enough of the terrifying hallucinations that you knew came from the drug.

Our friends Hanne and Ole, who we always went to the Skagen Festival with, clearly remember the time six months before when we visited you at St. Hans Hospital and were out for a walk with you in the beautiful grounds. Suddenly you pointed up a tree and screamed, 'Look, up in the tree, all those arms and legs dripping with blood!'

You ran back to the ward terrified. We followed and told the staff about your gruesome experience, which we couldn't understand because you were taking medicine that was supposed to counter-act hallucinations.

The staff told us you were feeling much better. This surprised us, of course, since not even in our wildest dreams could we imagine anything worse than seeing bloody body parts hanging in trees.

You would not return to the hospital, and three days later you were officially considered discharged. So for the next half year you were based at home and drug-free.

You were doing much better than you had during the previous nine months of hospitalization.

Physical distress such as vomiting, dizziness and strange mouth movements quickly moderated and soon disappeared complete-ly. Most importantly, your creepy and distressing hallucinations stopped completely.

But something had happened to you since your drug poisoning and your first encounter with antipsychotic medication.

It was hard for me to put my finger on it. You could almost com-pare it to the time you were on epilepsy medication, when you became slightly irascible and muddled, and when you also had a tendency to isolate yourself.

You insisted a few times that your favorite pop idol, Bon Jovi, was your father.

You were certainly doing better than during your hospital stay but significantly worse than before you were admitted in the summer of 1992. It was obvious that the poisoning and the mas-sive chemical treatment had taken a heavy toll.

Children and adults with autism and Asperger's syndrome are particularly vulnerable to the long-term effects of medication given as a sedative, especially antipsychotics.
Tony Attwood

Luise, you could more or less handle daily chores like cooking and shopping. You had become more clear-headed and able to plan and accomplish things outside the house. But it was still quite different from the time I visited you in St. Hans Hospital when you could barely drag yourself out of bed. And you became more and more outgoing, as long as I didn't push you to go back to the hospital.

We planned a vacation in England. And you insisted we should go by bus on this trip rather than taking our usual North Sea ferry voyage from Esbjerg to Harwich. You had our last rough crossing in mind. I remember it well, too. We sailed into a storm and got seasick.

I also got proof on this trip that Ole Svendsen was right.

Your interest in art and history led us far and wide.

Luise had her favorite artists, whose paintings we always sought out in the different museums. These included El Greco, the landscape painter William Turner, and the 16th century Dutch painters Hieronymus Bosch and Pieter Brueghel.

Our friends Jenni, Nigel and Dziga, who we used to stay with in London, had moved to Cornwall. So the plan was to visit them there. We would first spend a few days in London, so we could once again look at 'our' works of art and historic places and in general enjoy the atmosphere of the English capital.

When we went Luise had been drug-free for three months.

The trip included a two-day stay at a youth hostel in Highgate in North London. We didn't have the address, just a phone number.

The bus ride through Northern Europe was arduous. The German motorways seemed endless. By way of consolation we stopped at many rest areas where we could take a break and stretch. We crossed on the ferry from Calais to Dover. As we sailed in at the crack of dawn, a beautiful sight revealed itself. The faint morning sunlight bathed the white cliffs, turning them slightly pink.

We both started singing, as if we'd been given a stage cue: 'There'll be blue skies over the white cliffs of Dover.' She sang and I hummed along. Luise knew the song from the choral evenings at Tvind. I was suddenly transported back to my childhood, sitting on the floor in front of the radio and listening to Vera Lynn's beautiful voice rising from behind the static.

When we docked on the English south coast we'd been awake for 24 hours. And we didn't get any sleep on the bus journey from Dover to London. We were too excited at being in our beloved England again. We enjoyed every moment, every passing scene. It was the first time we'd driven through Canterbury's narrow streets and past the beautiful cathedral. It was quite magnificent, seen from the top deck of the bus. Then we made our way along the narrow winding roads through the picturesque Kent countryside.

We arrived at London's Liverpool Street Station around noon. Now we had to find our hostel in North London, so we decided to take the Underground to Highgate.

From Liverpool Street Station we took a train to Tottenham Court Road, where we would change to the Northern Line for Highgate. The Northern Line lies very deep, so we took the escalator five levels down. The platform was thronged with people, with trains arriving and leaving every two minutes.

I forgot to tell Luise that the Northern Line divides into two routes, and we wouldn't be taking the first train. Then suddenly she was gone – she'd apparently jumped on the first train that came. Heavens above!

She had no address, no money on her, and was dead tired.

I panicked and immediately dashed up to the control room where they directed all Tube traffic.

They searched for her, without success.

Then I contacted the police and reported Luise missing. They were very understanding and concerned for her safety. They told me: 'London is a dangerous city for a young girl alone and without money.'

I rang Jenni several times to see if by any chance she'd shown up in Cornwall, but she hadn't. She didn't have a penny on her. But she'd always been good at finding her way around and her demeanor somehow inspired confidence, so she could easily have made a train journey after promising to pay for the ticket later.

Poor thing! She hadn't slept for a day and a half and hadn't eaten since six that morning.

At five o'clock the next morning the police arrived – with Luise, thank God! The constables couldn't come into the bunk room where I slept, as it was for women only. I wasn't allowed to go out. So Luise was handed over at the door and had to quietly slip into bed. She had only two hours to sleep – we had to be up at seven. She'd barely rested when we left the hostel with our luggage. It was a creepy, old-fashioned and unfriendly place, so we had no desire to spend another night there.

We popped over to nearby Highgate Cemetery to see Karl Marx's grave, before leaving North London for the city center to find more agreeable accommodation where she could get caught up on her sleep.

Luise did the one right thing when she realized she'd got on the train without me. She got off at the next station and waited for me to come. A very sensible course of action. After waiting for me in vain, she headed back to the station where we'd started, but I was up in the control room searching for her on all the trains. She wasn't on any train, because she'd got off at the next station. It was me that was confused and did the wrong thing. The bottom line was that she was now left entirely to own devices. The only thing she could do was wander around hoping to find me.

Luise endured 17 hours on the streets of London without money, so she couldn't even get anything to eat or drink.

I can't imagine how tired and hungry she must have been. But strangely enough, I was sure she'd somehow handle it.

Luise was good at learning from experience. She was quick-witted and cautious. She could sense which people she could safely approach and which to avoid.

She loved wandering around the London's West End, especially the bustling area around Carnaby Street.

Luise was actually found in Carnaby Street at 4.30 am. Carnaby Street has a really vibrant nightlife. It's possible she decided to head over there simply because she loved this street – at least, during daylight hours.

Luise later told me she'd got talking to some friendly people who took her out to eat. She'd spoken to several interesting people who wanted to help. She'd had an eventful day, but had clearly been worried about how the day might end.

Luise, as usual you handled yourself brilliantly – even in the midst of London's nightlife.

You would never have managed this if you'd been sedated with antipsychotic drugs.

Why didn't you contact the police? You were usually very competent at this sort of thing.

Maybe you had contacted the police, but at a point before my missing person report had got into the system.

Maybe you wanted to spend a day without me in your beloved London.

Maybe your resources had been compromised by the strong chemicals you'd been exposed to during the previous year.

These questions will remain unanswered forever.

26

Drugs and hallucinations

You medication dose was quickly increased.
Those horrid, gruesome hallucinations returned.
Once again you were back in the drug hell
you knew only too well.

In late October 1993 Luise was again admitted to the hospital.

She was found wandering around Copenhagen Airport late one evening. I know she loved to walk around there, soaking up that special cosmopolitan atmosphere and dreaming of traveling far away.

According to the police, Luise was roaming around the airport without luggage. They must have thought she needed help and picked her up. They said she was glad for the help.

And, of course, if you told them you were waiting for your father, the pop music icon Bon Jovi, I can't really blame them for calling the National Hospital's Ward O to see if they knew you. Which indeed they did.

Unfortunately, the police then drove you to the intake desk at the National Hospital's psychiatric unit.

According to the chart, the police said: 'When the patient realized we were driving her to the National Hospital, she started to yell.'

You were admitted to the psychiatric unit.

How I would wish they'd just driven you home.

The October 26 chart note says of your admission – for the one and only time in your 600-page thick chart – 'The patient did not appear hallucinatory, but has been easily aroused to verbal aggression when the talk turns to drug therapy.'

Of course you got angry when the talk turned to drugs. You knew from bitter experience that the drug treatment would give you the hallucinations that you knew only too well and hated. You may have been afraid you'd be poisoned again.

In the years since then I showed your various psychiatrists the chart notes from October 26, 1993, saying you were not hallucinating when admitted, after half a year without drugs. I hoped it would get them to see that you were better off without medication. And also get them to see that these hallucinations, which according to their record repeatedly indicated you were very ill, were actually generated by the medication. The psychiatrists gave it a casual glance and said, 'We don't believe it.'

It is heartbreaking to read the five pages of Luise's chart from the first two days after she was readmitted. There is little to suggest the doctors talked to her as a person. For example, it says: 'She has a registered address in Brumleby, but supposedly does not live there. At the time of writing it is uncertain when she was discharged from St. Hans Hospital or when the medication treatment ended.'

As if Luise didn't know she lived in Brumleby! Had the psychiatrist ever talked to her? She was so fond of that apartment, which she'd had for four years already. Maybe she tried to tell them that she stayed some of the time in our summer house in Kulhuse, which was also true. And wouldn't she have known how long she'd been off the medication? And when she absconded from St. Hans Hospital? The psychiatrist simply must not have asked Luise about any of the above.

The second day after her admission is written under the heading 'Objectively': 'The patient was found to be both alert and oriented during the morning and afternoon. But she has been easily aroused to verbal aggression when talk turns to drug therapy. She has not appeared to be hallucinatory, but has been wandering about somewhat and is slightly bewildered and little-girl-like in her behavior.'

> *It seems you had a few days on sedatives before they started with the antipsychotic medication. This happened on October 29, and with great reluctance on your part.*

> *On November 1 the tone gets sharper: 'We can no longer wait and see how the condition develops. The alternative is that the patient does not go along with her treatment and we probably have to mandate treatment. The patient spends a long time 'chewing it over,' then refuses to say anything. Then slightly upset, she asks why she must take the medication, and when I inform her that she is ill she becomes angry. She just sits there and finally the patient takes her medicine.'*

In the chart notes I see that after six months outside the walls Luise had come back to the hospital ward where she was hospitalized shortly after the drug poisoning, and where she clearly had a very hard time. Could the doctor not see how much better she now felt after being drug-free for an extended period?

At that time they had written that she was 'marked by very poor cognition.' This would certainly not have been an assessment of her on October 26.

The chart notes from the first days suggest that there was no two-way conversation, but that the psychiatrist just asked questions and Luise answered. It says nothing about what happened in the half year Luise spent at home. If this had been the case Luise would gladly have told stories about the past six months. About her time in Kulhuse, where she lived alone for an extended period and went for a walk every morning with the neighbor's dog Sniffer.

She would have told about our trip to England, walking in the rugged Cornwall countryside – she was the one who saved us when we got lost. With her gurgling laughter she would have told them about the time I insisted I'd found a 'shortcut' to Zennor. Even though she didn't agree, she still came along because I stubbornly insisted we were on the right track. Luise was right. We were way off track. Suddenly we were standing at the edge of a 300-foot cliff that dropped straight down to the raging Atlantic. She was laughing while she took a photograph of me standing by my 'shortcut' and she later wrote on the shot: 'Oops, looks like we took a wrong turn.'

Luise could have talked endlessly about all the good times she'd had during her six months without medication.

She could have mentioned she hadn't felt as good as she might wish, but at least had felt much better than when medicated, and that she absolutely did not want to go back to a state where, due to heavy drugging, she would again have hallucinations and be drained of all energy and initiative.

But no one took the time to hear how her last half year had gone. It seemed as though her time 'outside the walls' did not exist.

Luise was given no chance to tell why she did not want the medication. Instead, they just threatened her with forced drugging if she did not accept it. She was also told she needed the medication because she was very ill.

There is not much to hope when you're a psychiatric patient.

After a few days on the medication, the chart says: 'undoubtedly psychotic.' Now the dose was further increased to curb the psychosis (which she'd got from the medicine).

Oh, no! Luise had just begun to recover from the brain damage caused by the drug poisoning. And now it looked like it was going to start all over again.

I had been able to see how Luise was slowly getting better. Luise could feel it herself. When I think how nine months earlier she had acted like a baby, and the duty nurse at the hospital had believed she was totally incapacitated, it was now clear there had been significant improvement and she was making good progress.

If for example Luise had had a brain hemorrhage, you would naturally expect rehabilitation and allow plenty of time before she could feel anything like her old self.

But such is not the case when the brain caves in after being poisoned with psychotropic drugs.

On November 15, 1993, the medicine had 'worked.' Now Luise was back in the old tormented state. She is described as psychotic, tormented, muddled and anxious.

Four days later: 'At intervals the patient screams and shows severely regressed behavior. She has told staff that she harbors very macabre images of knives, blood and murder.'

All these gruesome images were naturally seen as indicating an evolution of the illness, and now to top it off they started with the really heavy medication, and Luise again reached the point where she was so drugged that she could not resist.

The chances of being treated normally are very slim once you're diagnosed with schizophrenia. It seems that all behavior and every word uttered must be interpreted as symptoms of this disorder.

If you don't want to take antipsychotic medication because you get overwhelmed by the side-effects, this indicates lack of compliance, i.e. the patient does not agree to follow the prescribed treatment or medication. This in turn is viewed as a typical sign of a disorder in the psychosis spectrum.

If you find that you get worse from the drug and therefore raise questions about why you should take it, then you lack insight about your illness, which is also characteristic of individuals suffering from serious psychiatric disorders.

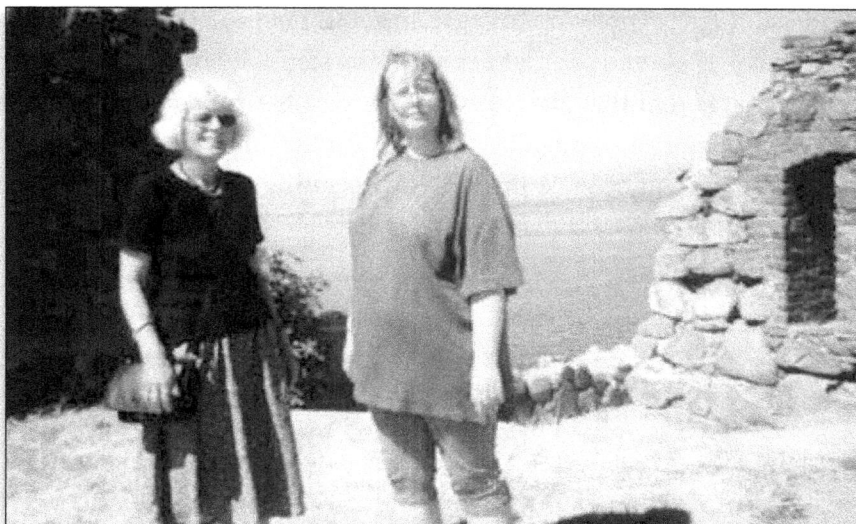

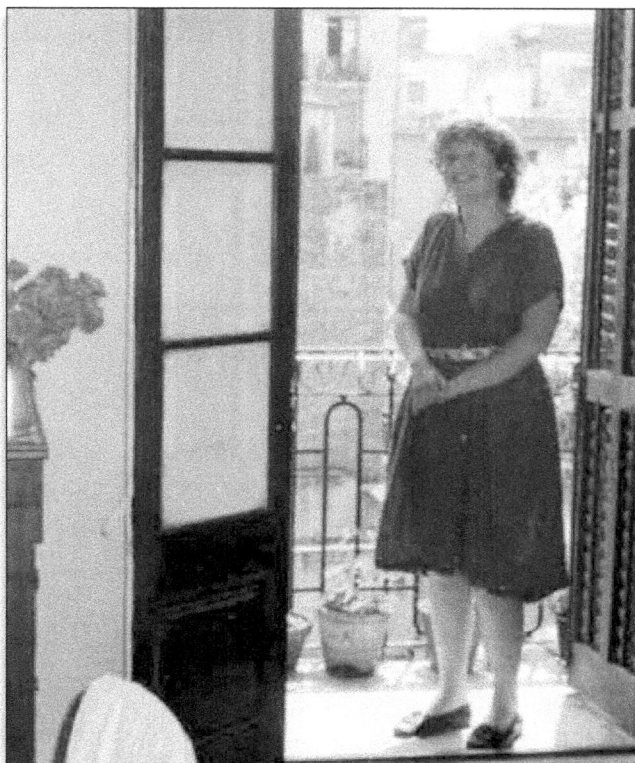

With Mom in Hammershus; on a balcony in Barcelona.

Luise said she threw up because she could not tolerate the medicine. The psychiatrists could see that her vomiting stemmed from a mental condition. She was told that she threw up because her subconscious rejected the medicine and responded by getting rid of it this way. As psychiatrist Finn Jørgensen might have put it: 'The vomiting was a sign of internal psychological processes that in turn was caused by her condition.'

In any other therapeutic discipline vomiting would immediately be interpreted as a sign that the patient could not tolerate the medication, and appropriate treatment would be administered.

People with psychiatric diagnoses are rarely taken seriously when they complain about physical symptoms, which might include chest pains, extreme exhaustion, or worse. Their complaints are often disregarded and interpreted as being psychologically triggered. During one hospital stay Luise sprained her ankle. It is noted in several places that she had a sore ankle and had difficulty putting any weight on her foot. The injury was never investigated, just noted in her chart under the heading of 'usual physical complaints'. Ten years later it emerged there had been a fracture that had mended crookedly.

On January 3, 1994, Luise was transferred to St. Hans Hospital.

27

PARANOID SCHIZOPHRENIA

The patient appears to be hallucinating.
The patient seems to hear voices.
The patient seems distressed.

On February 11, 1994, Luise was diagnosed with schizophrenia.

Luise became a 'schizophrenic' within two hours of being admitted to the National Hospital.

What happened was that on February 8 she again absconded from the National Hospital and came home to me.

I well remember your arrival home. It was very strange. You could hardly stand on your feet. You sat down, threw up all over the place, and then fell into a deep sleep that lasted for hours.

As soon as you woke up, I immediately started trying to persuade you to return to the hospital. I tried to convince you of how dangerous it could be to suddenly stop the medication. And you hadn't brought your pills home with you.

You would not go back. You got mad at me, went over to your own apartment and locked yourself in.

You never told me the reason why you ran away. I first learned this later from your chart – for three weeks you'd been strapped down and forcibly medicated. You had simply had enough.

Had I known this, I would have better understood your decisive response.

I was visiting you during the three weeks you'd been strapped down, but no straps were visible during visiting hours, so I didn't have a clue.

You ran home, where, oblivious of what you'd been through, I asked you to go back to 'your hell.'

Why wasn't I allowed to know that you'd been strapped down?

No wonder you often felt I didn't help you.

Now I understand your reaction, why you went to your apartment and locked yourself in.

I now know your anger was a reaction to my wanting to send you back to the appalling conditions you'd just escaped from.

But I got scared when you wouldn't open your door for me during the next three days.

I saw your anger and rejection as a product of your desperation. I was petrified at the thought that you might try to take your own life for a third time in the 18 months you had spent at St. Hans Hospital.

Our family doctor, who knew of your previous suicide attempts, couldn't get you to open the door either. She suggested forced hospitalization.

I must admit I was relieved at this proposal, because I was afraid of losing you, my sweet.

The doctor phoned the National Hospital, and you were admitted with 'yellow papers,' the procedure used when it is thought the chances of improvement would deteriorate markedly without in-patient treatment.

Luise was picked up by the police after lunch and taken to the National Hospital. The officers were friendly. They came back and told me everything had gone calmly.

Luise was at the hospital for at most two hours before being transferred to St. Hans Hospital. Yet the psychiatrist could write two and a half pages of chart notes about what she supposed had happened. She could have asked Luise, or me, or Luise's doctor, but she failed to do any of this.

The two pages of chart notes resulted in Luise being diagnosed with a very serious condition – paranoid schizophrenia.

According to the chart, 'Diagnosis at admission: paranoid psychosis.'

The same day two hours later: 'Diagnosis at discharge: paranoid schizophrenia.'

I will try to shed light on how easily one can be stigmatized by a diagnosis that can never be erased from one's paperwork. In Luise's case, as far as I can see, it happened in the absence of any real conversation between her and the psychiatrist.

For example, it says in the chart: 'As far as we know, the patient was found by the police.' The psychiatrist surely must have known that Luise was picked up by the police in her apartment by arrangement with her doctor.

Regarding her medical history, the chart says, 'Medical history cannot be detailed. The patient has a toothache and overall body pains, but doesn't wish to talk about it.'

Later it says: 'Badly compromised contact capability, both formal and emotional. Seems tormented by her condition, appears hallucinatory, looking for things in the street. Looks as if she's hearing voices. Appears to be severely psychotic.'

This may well be a competent description of someone who is severely mentally ill. But it is just a standard description that most likely appears in all the medical records of patients diagnosed with schizophrenia or psychosis.

It was clear from the chart note that the only thing Luise had said during this short stay was that she had toothache and body pains. The rest was the psychiatrist's assumptions about how she felt.

If the psychiatrist had tried to talk with Luise, she would have learned why Luise had run away from St. Hans Hospital, namely because she had been forcibly medicated and strapped in her bed for 20 straight days.

The psychiatrist could have learned when Luise had run away, and then known how long she had been without medication. The psychiatrist did not know and apparently never investigated what medication Luise normally took. So she gave Luise a random dose of four different antipsychotic drugs plus sedatives. Among the four preparations were Cisordinol, from which Luise had already been seriously poisoned and therefore should not be taking.

To me it's very disturbing that care providers, the very people who should be alert to the effects of these strong brain medicines, go handing them out like candy. This is the exact opposite of what the Board of Health regulations stipulate. The rule makes it clear that you only administer one antipsychotic at a time. However, it is acceptable to administer two drugs if there are well-documented reasons.

When Luise returned to St. Hans Hospital, they put her in a different ward from the one she had fled. In the new ward, they didn't know what medicine Luise had been on at the National Hospital or in the other ward, so she was again given four new, powerful anti-psychotic drugs. This meant that within five days her medication had radically changed three times. It is not very reassuring that doctors are so blasé about these dangerous drugs.

Luise, through all these years you've personally experienced psychiatrists prescribing antipsychotic drugs far too casually. You've always been given more prescriptions at a time, and in larger doses, than recommended. When you still felt bad after a heavy dosing, they just added a little more medication. The medical specialists never seemed to consider the fact that you got worse from the side-effects of large doses of medication, and therefore should have the dosage reduced rather than increased.

Luise's diagnosis was 'paranoid schizophrenia' after this two-hour stay at the National Hospital on February 11.

A brief stay that generated plenty of guesswork about your presumed hallucinations.

A stay where they guessed wrong about what had happened in the days before your admission.

A stay where they wrote up the classic standard description of a schizophrenic.

It does not seem important to the specialists that their chart notes are correct. On the other hand, it is important that something is written down that demonstrates they have 'rendered service.'

The chart is the authoritative document about a patient. If it is enshrined in the record that a person is schizophrenic, it is incontrovertible, whether right or wrong.

A psychiatrist may at any time – and apparently without talking to the patient – issue a diagnosis that can have dire consequences in the patient's future life. This is rather unsettling.

The sad thing is simply that this slipshod handling of cases happens all too often, according to what I have since heard from other people.

28

COMMITTED FOR TREATMENT

More mentally ill sentenced to compulsory treatment.
Total committed for treatment increasing every year.
From 2004 to 2006 the total rose by up to 35%.

Headlines from Danish newspapers

A sentence to undergo psychiatric treatment is a specific measure a court can impose on a mentally ill defendant in place of the usual criminal punishment. Criminally insane, or psychotic, offenders are legally absolved from penalty, if the court – usually after psychiatric evaluation and an opinion from the legal medical council – finds the defendant to be insane at time of the offense. In cases of less severe mental illness, the court may sentence a defendant to treatment to prevent future criminal activity. This can be repealed by a new ruling.

This special measure is meant to protect the mentally ill who commit serious crimes and who need the kind of treatment for their condition that is not possible in an ordinary prison.

The problem is that treatment sentences are handed out too liberally, and often at the practitioner's discretion, as Peter Kramp, chief physician at the National Hospital's clinic for court-ordered psychiatry, said in 2007: 'If a psychiatrist believes that a person needs prolonged hospitalization, a treatment sentence may well be recommended, even though the criminal behavior is not that extreme. It's simply medical discretion.'

This means that a minor criminal offense committed by a person with a psychiatric diagnosis may lead to committal, if the doctor thinks the culprit needs treatment and recommends it. The concept of a fair trial does not apply to this group of people. This is what Luise had to go through at St. Hans Hospital.

In April 1994 Luise was smoking in bed, as she often did. That day – I believe by mistake – she had been given an extra large dose of Nozinan, a strong sedative antipsychotic. Luise fell asleep with her cigarette burning and the bedclothes caught fire. The watch nurse spotted the blaze and quickly extinguished it, but the incident sparked a long and humiliating legal process that ended with Luise getting an indefinite treatment sentence. Everyone knew that the comforter had caught fire because Luise had fallen asleep holding a lit cigarette. Yet she got dragged through a legal case she did not have a fair chance of winning. The sentence was handed down on the basis of a written opinion from a physician who did not know Luise. The staff who knew Luise was never asked anything. Luise received an indefinite sentence, which in effect could last a lifetime, for falling asleep with a cigarette.

In May 1997 I wrote an article for the Danish magazine, *Mind*. It was about Luise's trial and carried the headline 'Well, at least we don't burn witches anymore.' It describes a 'completely ordinary case' against a seriously mentally ill patient.

On June 18, 1996, Luise faced the court in Roskilde in a deep psychotic state. She was charged with arson. A custodian and a defense attorney had been appointed for her.

When you look at the court proceedings and read the 'indictment' and 'court record,' it looks like a totally unremarkable case.

Excerpts from the indictment: 'In violation of Penal Code paragraph 181, Luise is accused of setting fire to her bedding in the locked ward of St. Hans Hospital, where she was a patient.' Then: 'The judgment of the court is that the accused be sentenced to treatment at the mental hospital with supervision by the probation service following discharge.'

The court record states: 'The accused has pleaded guilty and has given evidence.' Later it says: 'The court considers it expedient, in order to prevent further offenses, that the measures recommended by the prosecution be implemented.' So it really is happening! She gets a mandatory treatment sentence.

It is true that Luise pleaded guilty to arson, but she pleaded guilty to a lot of things, including killing all her children (she never had any) and selling drugs in the U.S. (she had never been to the U.S. before 1997, nor had anything to do with drugs). She kept on pleading guilty, I have been told, until she threw up in the courtroom, after which the trial was concluded. She didn't get burned at the stake, like in medieval times, but this legal process was an anxiety-provoking and humiliating experience for her.

Luise now had papers showing she was a criminal sentenced to mandatory treatment. She had never before had any contact with the criminal justice system, and she had only had contact with police when they took her to the hospital when she was considered a danger to herself.

Protected in the locked ward? These patients, many hospitalized because they are a danger to themselves, are apparently also a danger to themselves after they are admitted to a secure unit. Furthermore, if they commit a 'crime' while in hospital they are then subject to the normal procedures of police interrogation. One might wonder what kind of truth the police can arrive at when interviewing a severely psychotic person. Is it really the sort of 'truth' that can form the basis for a trial?

As for the court's decision – 'sentenced to treatment at the mental hospital ... in order to prevent further offences' – Luise was supposedly in the safest place, at a mental hospital, when the offense occurred.

In short, I think this trial and procedures leading up to it are a disgrace to the Danish legal system, which needs to be addressed in parliament. It cannot be right that the mentally ill actually do not have the same rights as other citizens.

Luise's case was unfortunately not an isolated incident, as I learned after my article appeared in *Mind*. I subsequently got several reports about mentally ill patients who, like Luise, were sentenced to mandatory treatment for minor offenses.

In 2005 a report was published by the Institute for Human Rights, which also stated that the meting out of treatment sentences lacks proportionality. Minor offenses, which for the non-mentally ill lead to dropped charges, a fine or brief imprisonment, can set in motion extended treatment sentences with possible mandatory hospitalization.

Luise treatment sentence was rescinded in 1998, but she would never get rid of the label of arsonist.

I see from Luise's journal that, shortly before she died, the cigarette incident was brought up again. By then more than 11 years had passed since it happened. The psychiatrist pointed to the mandatory treatment sentence to show how dangerous she was. This criterion of danger was supposed to justify giving Luise a second antipsychotic on top of the drugs she was already taking – chart note dated July 4, 2005: 'It must be remembered that the patient has repeatedly been aggressive and a danger to herself and others. She has been responsible for an incident of arson.'

The psychiatrist got his message across. Nobody could then be in any doubt how dangerous Luise should be considered, and how important it was that she got the increased medication – with fatal consequences.

29

A FIVE-MINUTE CONSULTATION

The psychiatrist did not know Luise.
Talked with her for five minutes,
misunderstood her, and the result was
a heavier dose of medication.

On September 22, 1995, Luise finally got a place in the Sundbygård psychiatric nursing home, a center housing 200 residents in 12 living units.

Luise got a room in Unit 5. Her new accommodation measured roughly 9 x 12 ft., quite small considering she paid the full rate. But that was a minor problem, since she now finally had her own place. There were also pleasant shared facilities, including a lounge, communal kitchen and three bathrooms. Each washing/toilet facility was for 20 residents. The staff was dedicated and made much of the idea that the residents should feel they were all one big family. The place's history was that it had been a nursing home for senile patients and was now in the process of closing down, so as rooms became available mental patients were moved in. When Luise got there, most of the residents suffered from senile dementia.

> *It was such a relief that you could now be in your own bed. You could sit in your own chair and listen to the music you wanted to hear on the radio without anyone coming in to change the station. You could even choose what you wanted to watch on television. All those creepy experiences from St. Hans Hospital – waking up to a fire in your bed, forcible injections with syringes, being strapped down – you could put behind you, at least during the daytime. But problems remained. Your nights were filled*

with horrible nightmares. I saw this when I stayed overnight with you in Unit 5 and also when you were home in Brumleby.

You especially had two kinds of recurring nightmares. One was that your bed had caught fire. You would wake up screaming and drenched in sweat. When you were yourself again, you could tell me about it. The other theme of your nightly horror show was that doctors were holding you down and sticking needles in you. Shivers run down my spine when I remember one particular nightmare. You were screaming and gesticulating wildly. It was almost impossible to get you out of this terrible state. You dreamed that Kurt, a doctor from St. Hans, was bent over you. As you related: 'Kurt's head was huge and right in my face, and he had a very large syringe in his hand that he was going to stick in me, and he said with a wicked grin in a husky voice that nobody would ever know. He was going to stick the syringe into my brain, Mom.'

It was a dream you couldn't get out of your body. I was there to see your reaction only once, but I could understand from you that it was a recurring nightmare.

Unfortunately you spent most of the days in your new home fast asleep in bed. No wonder, as the mega-dose of medicine they gave you at St. Hans Hospital followed you to your new location.

From Luise's moving into Unit 5 and over the next five years, there were five different consulting psychiatrists loosely attached to the place. But there was a permanent medical director, who had overall responsibility and who seemed to have a good sense of what his patients needed. There were very few patient conferences with you, but the psychiatrists sometimes consulted with staff members. I knew from your caregivers that the staff had always believed that you received too much medication. They had been aware of your vomiting and could see you felt better after throwing up the medicine, having absorbed less of it.

There is not a single chart note where vomiting is not seen as a problem, but the psychiatrists never associated it with Luise's inability to tolerate the medication, although I know the staff mentioned this at every opportunity. The psychiatrists were aware that Luise was overwhelmed by the heavy medication, and I see that questions were being raised about why she was getting a large dose of Trileptal (an antiepileptic drug), along with the antipsychotic, when she didn't have epilepsy.

This antiepileptic was discontinued in early January 1997. Chart note from February 26, 1997: 'The patient has become more awake and lively since the Trileptal was discontinued. Reduction of Rivotril (clonazepam) dose will now also be tried.'

Further dose reductions were occasionally considered, but were never really implemented, perhaps because the psychiatrist who had prescribed it would soon be replaced by a new psychiatrist, who in turn would just wait and see. The problem was that the consulting psychiatrists were in-house for too a short a time to implement a long-term plan to reduce the dose.

In January 1998 I managed to arrange a conference with the consultant psychiatrist at the time, whom I told about the drug poisoning Luise had suffered at St. Hans Hospital. I also expressed my concern about the heavy drug doses she was being given. He agreed she was getting a lot of medication and said they would continue discussing this. It is on record that I thought she was taking too much medicine, but unfortunately there was no mention that this problem should be addressed.

I notice that several of the consultants never got to meet Luise, so it was mostly about paperwork rather than actual face time, but they did their best under the circumstances, and after the few times they did talk with her she was described positively – that is, as a person rather than a diagnosis. For instance, they wrote that she was friendly and smiling and had positive relationships with staff and residents, and she had no problems taking the medication. Luise was not good in large groups but was caring and loving towards residents who were troubled, so she was well liked and respected in the care home. Luise did have special abilities.

A patient called Thea often phoned and told me about Luise. She described Luise as a wonderful girl capable of spreading happiness and wellbeing. One time, when Thea had shut herself in her room because she felt miserable, Luise came in to her and sang '*Che sera, sera,*' then she danced and entertained Thea until she was finally in a good mood again. Thea will never forget her for that. Luise was also the only person who could calm residents who flipped out. One time I was there in Unit 5 when Niels ran amok. Niels was a big guy, and most residents were afraid of him because he could suddenly turn very angry and aggressive. Nobody knew when or why it might happen.

We were all sitting together in the living room one day, when suddenly ominous sounds could be heard coming from the kitchen – angry yelling, kitchenware thrown around, a table overturned, a chair smashed. The caregiver who had been involved in the disturbance walked into the room shaken. There was a dead silence from residents and staff. I was also shaken when Niels suddenly burst into the living room, dark with rage. Now what was going to happen? Well, Luise stood up, went over to Niels, put her arm on his shoulder and said, 'Come on, Niels, let's go to my room, smoke a cigarette and relax.'

Niels went with her. I wonder what would have happened if Luise had not been present. One thing is certain. Niels was beyond the reach of the trained caregivers. The staff told me afterwards: 'It's strange, but Luise is the only one who can reach Niels when he gets himself into a corner. It must be because she's not afraid of him.' As an aside to myself, I could add, 'and because he can sense that she likes him.'

I can see from notes of the few meetings Luise had with the psychiatrists that they talked to her as a person. They had time to listen and reach an understanding that the muddled start Luise often made to a conversation was due to nervousness. They had to get past this, and then the conversation would become quite normal.

Luise met with the psychiatrist in April 1998. Among issues dis-cussed was the treatment sentence from 1994 that was still in force. She began as usual with her confused chatter but gradually became more articulate, and the psychiatrist concluded from the conversation that he thought it quite unlikely that she had started a fire on purpose, because she seemed to be afraid of fire. Staff at Luise's care home had said the same.

The psychiatrist's intervention got the ball rolling to finally rescind the indefinite treatment sentence from 1994.

April 8, 1998:
'The situation is thoroughly discussed with staff members (in Unit 5), who have known Luise throughout her stay, and the conclusion is that she poses no risk of dangerous behavior.'
Chart note from June 10, 1998:
'Query from the Police Chief in Roskilde asking whether it is appro-priate to continue enforcing the court-ordered measure to prevent further offenses. Statement attached from St. Hans Hospital, April 16, 1997 ... It was determined that the risk of further offences of this nature were extremely slim, with a recommendation that the court order be lifted. However, the public prosecutor decided against this course of action.'

As it turned out, it would take over a year and a half and endless pa-perwork from the time of the first recommendation to revoke the man-datory treatment sentence until this was actually achieved.

On November 25, 1998, Luise's treatment sentence was lifted after a long hard slog. It had been much easier to hand out the sentence than to lift it. It was all over in half an hour at an ostensibly normal hear-ing without any preliminaries or witnesses. The decision was based on a piece of paper written by a psychiatrist, who as far as I could tell did not know Luise. His words were incontrovertible, so there was no reason to proceed according to normal rules.

Luise's drug intake was scaled back somewhat in the first year, but both I and the caregivers thought this should have happened much faster. I made a written request on March 21, 1999, for a conference with the psychiatrist, which Luise's contact person should also attend. I can see from the chart that I also wrote that I thought Luise threw up because she could not tolerate the heavy medication.

The chief physician approved my request and wrote a note on April 6, 1999, saying: '... It is especially important to expand contact with Luise's mother, who in her case is a resource person.'

The family conference was finally set up for June 11. A half hour was allotted. Luise's contact person, Lise, and I both showed up well prepared. Lise was a nurse and the care home's assistant director. Our only goal was to get Luise's medication dose reduced. We had already agreed that Lise would take the lead. She put forth strong arguments for why she felt Luise's dosage should be reduced. She said that Luise received very high doses of medication and yet still had hallucinations. And that Luise slept most of the day for the same reason. Might it not be a good idea to try reducing the dose for a time and see how it works out?

I asked if it was possible the medicine was making her hallucinate, since she had never been hallucinatory before starting on the antipsychotic drugs. The response to this was that it was unthinkable that the medication could cause hallucinations. This was only the case with opiates and Valium (Valium belongs to the same group as clonazepam, which Luise had taken). Luise had to be wakened and brought in for the last five minutes of the meeting. First, Luise wanted to know what we had talked about. Then she was asked how she was doing. Luise said she got scared at night because Martin from Unit 6, whose room was above hers, sent evil thoughts down to her. The psychiatrist looked serious and said it was evidence of 'thought transference.'

Both Lise and I both explained that Martin was often plagued by voices around midnight. He would start clattering with furniture and yell very harsh things like: 'Get out of here – I'll kill you!' I had heard

Martin's nocturnal rampage and could confirm that it was scary to be wakened like that.

But the psychiatrist did not even hear this. The record of the conference ends with: 'The patient was also informed that we talked about her medication, and that, based on her experiences (Martin sending evil thoughts), it would be wrong to reduce her dosage, and indeed an increased dose of Leponex (clozapine) might be considered. Both the patient and her mother accept this.'

In a page and a half of notes there is no mention of Lise's and my arguments for reducing Luise's medication dose. It is not even mentioned that Lise was present at the meeting. The record told otherwise. It is an evasion of the truth to say we agreed to increased medication for Luise – this was an edict.

30

MORE OF THE SAME

*The psychiatrist provides continuous specialist assistance
to care home residents in accordance with individual residents' needs.
This task is carried out in close cooperation with the residents,
the contact person and/or the unit's director.*

**From the contract between the County
and Copenhagen Hospital Corporation.**

Now we could see the light at the end of the tunnel. From January 2001 a psychiatrist from Amager Hospital was permanently attached to Sundbygård. It was almost too good to be true. An in-house specialist might finally think your high doses of medication should be continuously monitored. The psychiatrist started his new job by introducing himself as Sofus to each of the residents.

You liked him. He inspired confidence. You were sure that everything would be better with him. He would understand that you couldn't tolerate all that medicine, which was what caused you to throw up.

I was present when you first met with him. It went really well. He listened to you but said we just had to wait and see. He wanted to know you a little better before he started changing things. It sounded quite reasonable, and you felt reassured.

This turned out to be premature. You dosage was not reduced, as you had hoped. Quite the opposite, it was increased considerably. The worst thing was that he changed both the drugs and the dose far too often.

In 2003 I made a list of all the different drugs you'd been given after he became your doctor. You could also see how often the doses changed. In the first two years that Sofus was your psychiatrist you were given 11 different antipsychotic drugs (not including benzodiazepines) and doses went up or down 26 times.

I showed Sofus my overview. He could easily have checked whether I had got it right, because I included dates and referred to page numbers in the chart. But Sofus would not even look at my list.

Why are changes in medication so dangerous?

I'll try to give a simplified explanation. We know that antipsychotic drugs affect the brain's neurotransmitter system. Scientists have discovered that people with schizophrenia have an overproduction of or hypersensitivity to the neurotransmitter dopamine, which is found in different biochemical variants. It is believed that this overproduction/hypersensitivity needs to be limited before a person with schizophrenia can get any better. Various antipsychotic drugs have been developed that affect these variants in different ways and to varying degrees. That is partly what differentiates one product from another.

It is also well documented that a drug's effects are not evident for at least 14 days, and for certain preparations it can take up to a year before the maximum effect is apparent. That's why it's so dangerous to change medication or dosage as often as was the case for Luise. There is very little scientific evidence to show how different antipsychotics work together, but in practice people often get three or four antipsychotics simultaneously, because psychiatrists don't know what to do. It's fairly easy to figure out that everything in the brain may be partially put out of action, if it's true that each product has different ways of working.

We had previously thought your stalled treatment was due to always being treated by different psychiatrists who didn't know you. All the psychiatrists saw your vomiting as a problem. They were also amazed that you were still hallucinating despite the fact that your combined medication doses were far above the maximum recommended. But there

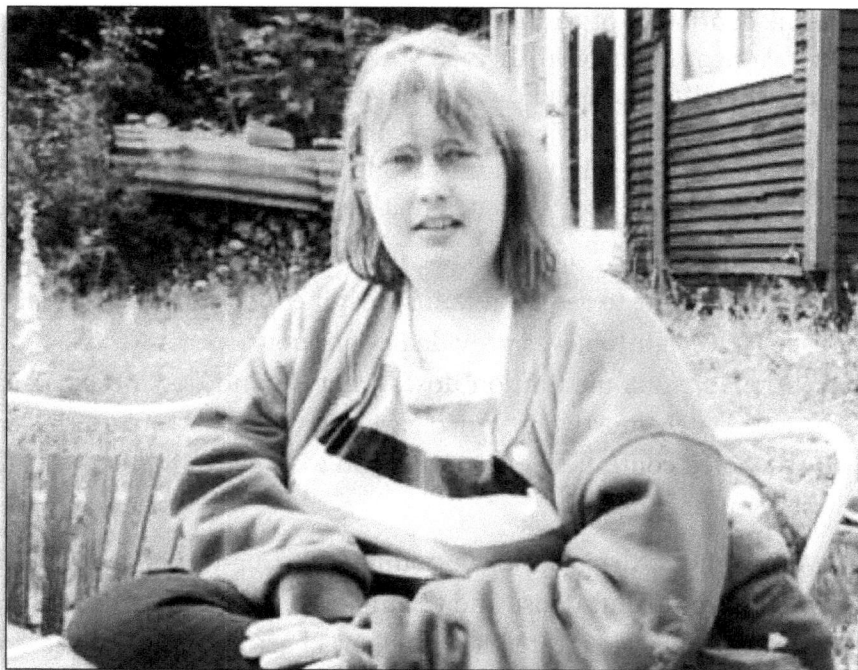

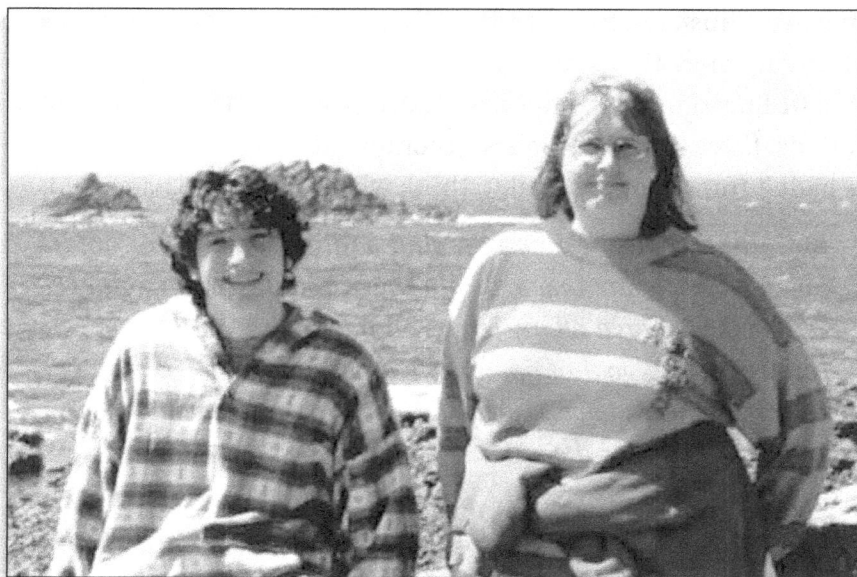

At the summer house in Kulhuse; with Dziga at Land's End, Cornwall.

was some continuity of treatment, since with few exceptions you always got the same amount of medicine. Now that you finally had a permanent psychiatrist, it seemed our hope for a stable, long-term treatment plan with a dosage reduction might become a reality. Instead, everything went haywire. It was surely not unreasonable to try reduced medication when there was plenty of evidence that heavy doses had not made you better, but rather the opposite.

It's hard for me to see what Sofus imagined his consultant position entailed. He certainly never provided continuous specialist assistance. As mentioned, your medication doses went up and down incessantly, and unfortunately mostly up, which gave you the most trouble. This can hardly be called continuity. For a while you were getting three times the highest recommended dose.

Antipsychotic drug dosage amounts are usually divided into the starting dose, a medium dose and the highest recommended dose. Professor Jes Gerlach has created an excellent chart of antipsychotic dosages, showing how, using a given conversion factor, multiple drugs doses can be administered together. But Gerlach points out that as far as possible giving more than one drug at a time should be avoided. In November 2001 Luise got four antipsychotic drugs at once, which corresponded to almost three times the highest recommended dose. This is fatal, and if she hadn't thrown up, I dread to think what might have happened.

Everything that you, I and the staff had said about your not being able to tolerate the medication was totally lost on Sofus. He completely ignored all my letters on the subject. So much for the county's stated goal of appointing a permanent consultant psychiatrist to work in close cooperation with the residents, the contact person and/or the unit's director.

Sofus went ahead with his own very questionable treatment, which resulted in Luise becoming a revolving-door patient at Amager Hospital's psychiatric ward. From early 2001 to May 2003 she was admitted 14 times.

Things always looked the same before you were admitted to hos-

*pital – either increased medication or vomiting. You would throw
up all the drugs over several days. Your mental state slowly improved, things got clearer. I noticed that you usually lost 20-25 lbs
in the process. After three to five weeks you were detoxified. This
meant that you kept down the next heavy drug dose, which acted
as an 'overdose' because the vomiting had flushed all medication
out of your system in the weeks before. So you slowly became
more and more hallucinatory and distressed. After three to four
weeks you felt so bad that you had to be hospitalized.*

*Your sense that you couldn't tolerate the medication was cor-
rect, but this didn't help when Sofus had a different opinion. He
believed that you had deteriorated because your condition had
taken a turn for the worse. He came up with psychological explanations, one such being that it's very common for mentally
ill people who don't recognize their illness to vomit in order to
avoid medical treatment. Therefore vomiting was just part of the
progression of your illness. And this could only be alleviated with
more medicine.*

*I could not accept the explanation that all this was due to psy-
chological causes, to the progression of your mental illness. I got
increasingly desperate and wrote to Sofus asking for a referral to
another psychiatrist for a second opinion, so fresh eyes could as-
sess your treatment.*

Sofus sent the following reply dated March 6, 2003:
'... I think it will be difficult to find a psychiatrist who would be
willing to make such an evaluation ... If a psychiatrist were to
review the process, his conclusion might well be that your daughter
is very ill, with perhaps a few details about the medication, so that
he could focus more on how you feel about your daughter's mental
illness. If such a psychiatric evaluation (of Luise's treatment) were
similar to my position, I'm not sure it would change anything, but

it would be more a question of whether you trusted the psychiatrist. If his evaluation were materially different from mine, I would
of course take it into consideration, though I cannot promise to
follow it – as long as I am responsible for the treatment I also
want a free hand. This situation would be extremely inopportune
for our future collaboration. And it would not really benefit Luise.'

We continue to break new ground in medical research. Hopefully, these advances can make drug treatments for mental disorders more targeted. In January 2003 I read an article in a psychiatry journal about a new research project at St. Hans Hospital. The idea was that people can now be tested for how their cytochrome P450 (CYP) liver enzymes metabolize psychotropic drugs. The theory assumes that if you have a slow conversion rate, which 7-10% of the population has, the medicine will accumulate in the body and cause side-effects.

I contacted the hospital's research team leader and told him about Luise's drug treatment and her vomiting. According to him, she should obviously be tested, as her liver enzymes probably produced a lower conversion rate, judging from the way she responded. As agreed, I sent the necessary papers and a list of Luise's medications to the research center in March 2003. Of course, I told Sofus about our plan and was confident he would think it was a great idea. Such a test might explain why Luise could not tolerate the medication.

On March 20 at 6:30 pm my phone rang. I was not there to take the call, but there was a message for me to call the research center urgently. I called and got the director on the phone. He talked non-stop for an hour and 18 minutes. He told me many times over that someone like Luise could not take the test because, even though the test might show she had poor drug absorption, it was still the psychiatrist's duty to prescribe this much medication with her being as ill as she was. I understand why he chose to call rather than write such nonsense. He was careful to add that, since I had now been informed, I would not be receiving a letter about the matter.

It is easy to figure out that Sofus was behind this response, because the research team leader said a lot of things about Luise that I had not briefed him on. My head was spinning after the long conversation, and I also felt very uneasy. I sat and mulled over this very strange phone call for a few days. Then I wrote a letter on March 24, asking for a written response to our request giving the reasons it was denied. I also wrote that I was amazed he had information about Luise not given by me. From what I had read about the research project, participation was completely anonymous.

My letter never received a reply.

31

A STORM OF ACCUSATIONS

*In the exercise of medical duties, a physician
has an obligation to exercise diligence,
including the cost-effective prescription of drugs,
use of assistants, etc.*

Article 272 of the 2001 law on medical practice

For several years now, I had been able to predict when Luise would be hospitalized, based on my observations of her throwing up and her reactions to drug dose increases. On February 3, 2003, Luise's dosage of the strong, slow-acting antipsychotic Orap (pimozide) was increased significantly. According to Jes Gerlach's conversion factor, she was at nearly twice the maximum recommended dose. Luise was hospitalized on April 8, 2003. The first day she was given the choice between an increased dose or being sent home. She reluctantly chose more medicine. Isn't that what we call veiled coercion?

After several days Sofus referred Luise for a long stay at St. Hans Hospital. She was terrified at the thought of going back there. Luise was very distressed and asked me to speak to the doctor on the ward. She hoped I could make it clear that she could not tolerate the medication and did not want to go to Roskilde. She knew from bitter experience that she would not be taken seriously.

I got an appointment at Amager Hospital on April 28. I was greeted by a shocking sight. Luise was hallucinating so much that she barely had time to hug me. She was running around wildly, trying to avoid the snakes and fictitious blood-soaked creatures that were coming out of the walls. She was also busy trying to protect me from them, pushing me around all over the place. A nurse who was on duty the last two nights told me this was the result of the last two drug dose increases.

One reason antipsychotic medicines are prescribed is to counteract hallucinations. Luise was now on twice the maximum recommended dose, which gave her the worst hallucinations imaginable. I did not understand the specialists. What were they thinking? I realize now that the psychiatrist, Elise, was somewhat uneasy about the situation. She was certainly very unpleasant towards both Luise and me.

When I walked into the interview room, she did not even look at me. She just leafed through chart notes, while throwing one accusation after another at me. For example, it was my fault Luise was not getting better because I was against the drug treatment. It was my influence that set Luise against going to St. Hans Hospital. The psychiatrist also recommended I stop visiting Luise on the grounds that, according to the staff, she felt bad after my visits. She went on and on, her head still buried in the chart. I don't remember us making eye contact even once. I never got the chance to ask questions about anything, since I had to defend myself against all the accusations.

The psychiatrist was now apparently planning to further increase your medication, so you had to be brought into the interview room. To put it mildly, she dragged you in, while you were still fighting off the terrifying apparitions. Suddenly Elise banged hard on the table and screamed: 'Stop it and sit down!' You obeyed, and then Elise asked, 'Do you want us to increase your medication?' You replied, 'I don't know.'

You were not mentally present at this meeting. But your medication was increased anyway.

The psychiatrist got your approval for an increased drug dosage. This is required by law and must be entered in a patient's chart. But was she treating you with due diligence?

Chart note from the same day: 'I speak with the patient, who urgently asks for more Seroquel (quetiapine), which is also indicated.'

You certainly did not urgently request more Seroquel. You had no idea what we were talking about. You were too busy dodging the bloodthirsty monsters coming out of the walls.

I wrote a letter to Elise after our conference, in which I pointed out that the staff would certainly not vouch for her claim that Luise felt worse after my visits – in fact, quite the opposite.

So I can ascertain that the chart note of this meeting was written after my letter. The note states: 'We recognize the importance of all parties working together on treatment, for the benefit of the patient, and the importance of regular contact between the patient and her mother, since the mother at one point assumed she was not wanted, an impression we seek to correct.'

The chart note from this conference is wrong. It gives the impression of an agreeable conversation in which I basically approve of the treatment. One gets the impression that Luise sits quietly and says she hears voices and urgently asks for more medicine.

The reality was unquestionably different.

32

COERCION AND REPRISALS

*Write on my gravestone that
it was the medication that killed me.*

Luise Hjerming Christensen, May 2003

You were terrified at the thought of returning to the St. Hans Psychiatric Hospital in Roskilde, where your whole sad story began, but there was no way around it. Sofus' argument for the decision was that the experts there would be able to find the right treatment for you.

The intention was good enough. But to get good results from this hospital stay it was essential to provide a detailed description of your problem.

This never happened.

Chart note on admission, dated April 16, 2003:
'A 30-year-old woman, very familiar to us, with schizophrenia and mental retardation. Being treated with Seroquel, Oxazepam, Clonazepam, Lyskantin, Orap and Stilnoct (zolpidem). The patient is resident at Sundbygård and over the past six months has repeatedly been admitted to Amager Hospital. Is distressed, hallucinatory and delusional, and her condition has been increasingly unstable in recent months. The patient is referred to St. Hans Hospital, as there is a need for hospitalization to stabilize her and adjust her medication. The patient gives her consent to this.'
Niels Hansen, junior doctor

The referral made it look like you'd only been hospitalized within the past six months and that you had worsened over the last two months. There was no mention that you had been a revolving-door patient for some three years. Not a word about the fact that you'd tried almost every antipsychotic medication – and in heavy doses. Your vomiting was not even mentioned. On the other hand, the referral letter pointed out that you were very willing to be hospitalized.

You were far from willing to be admitted when the note was written, and we tried everything to get the referral canceled. We should never have done that, for now the reprisals began. The form they took was that nobody would talk to us. Daytime staff was dismissive of you, administered all the extra medication you requested, of course, but otherwise made no positive contact. They were 'cold' towards you, as you put it. I sensed what you were talking about, because I was frozen out, to say the least, when I came to visit. The staff didn't even say hello. They turned their backs on me. Before, they had always been very welcoming.

Just a small example: while I was visiting you one day, you asked me to ask your nurse if they'd increased your medicine dose the previous day. The nurse sat alone in the courtyard with her feet up on a chair, reading a magazine. She hardly even looked up from her magazine, replying that she really didn't know. I was asking on your behalf, Luise, but your contact person would not answer the question. The situation was becoming really unpleasant for you, and now we had both become aware that St. Hans Hospital would be the lesser of two evils.

You were transferred in early May.

I've tried for myself to analyze Luise's chart notes. They present a very diverse picture. There are psychiatrists whose notes are highly relevant and clear-headed. Sadly, there are also some chart notes that leave me with a feeling that something that is not quite right is being covered up. This picture becomes clear when I read the notes dealing with the plan to transfer Luise to St. Hans Hospital. A lot of ink is used to tell how keen she is to go there and how much her mother tries to thwart this move.

Chart note dated April 16:

'The patient herself says she wants to move to St. Hans, as she needs a longer hospitalization and she is completely committed to this. Also says she is very distressed that her mother is interfering in her treatment and doesn't want us to tell her mother about the decision, because she is afraid of how her mother might react.'

I don't understand why such erroneous chart notes keep getting written. It clearly isn't to help the patient.

Your fear of returning to St. Hans stemmed from your previous dramatic experiences there.

I think it was after the April 16 conference, when Elise wrote in your chart that you so desperately wanted to get more medicine and move to St. Hans, that you started telling me: 'You can write on my gravestone that it was the medicine that killed me.' You would repeat this phrase frequently in the following months, and it made shivers run down my spine.

At St. Hans Hospital the first psychiatrist was shocked at the large doses of medication you had been getting at Amager Hospital and thoroughly reorganized your drug intake. Later a new psychiatrist came who again increased your medication, though nowhere near the dosage you'd been taking at Amager Hospital.

It was in February 2004 that your treatment took a turn for the better. I was called in for a conference about your treatment plan in early February. My sister Elsebeth came with me. We had agreed that Elsebeth would lead the discussion. She could ask the questions, as I knew from experience I would be fobbed off with the classic remark: 'It's hard for a mother to see her child so ill.' Said in a very emphatic tone, and with a strong hint that a mother is incapable of objectively evaluating her child's condition.

Elsebeth said she thought you were significantly worse after the last increase in medication. You were so bad that you barely had the energy to deal with our visit. The answer to this was that all the treatment team believed you had improved but it was probably too strenuous for you to have visitors.

I couldn't help saying, 'Does this mean you think Luise feels fine when she's so exhausted she can't even bother to see her family for half an hour four times a week? I grant you that she's not too much trouble for the staff, but it can't be right that this is a criterion for feeling fine. Compare this to six months before, when she got less medication and was full of life at the Skagen Festival. She was so excited at all the wonderful music that she stayed up until midnight every day.' The thing about less medicine was right in the sense that she'd thrown it all up, which has the same effect.

It was a great outing at Skagen. Best of all you liked to walk around the festival alone and talk to people. One adventure was your long chat with an Australian band. They bought you a soda in the big hall. You told me afterwards you thought their English accent was a bit funny. That was also the evening we finished with a nice fish supper at Brøndums Hotel.

The record of the two-hour long meeting in February was boiled down to: 'The staff feels that the patient has been doing much better, the family quite the opposite.'

At the big conference table sat a woman who did not participate in the discussion. She was there as your future psychiatrist. She took me aside after the meeting and with great interest asked about your life, Luise. She was clearly very surprised to hear that you could be a fully functional girl, because she certainly did not get that impression on first meeting you.

I talked and talked about you, my lovely Luise. About our exciting backpacking trip to America in 2001, when we traveled by Greyhound bus, and about all your hopes and dreams. I also managed to tell her that the times you felt best were when you threw up most of your medicine, becoming more or less drug-free. I told her that during all your years on medicine you'd been pronounced mentally retarded and, if I hadn't found out in time and said no, you would have been transferred to a home for the mentally retarded. I knew it was the medication that slowed down your thinking so much that you appeared to be retarded.

In March 2004 the new psychiatrist took over your treatment. She treated you like a human being, not some impersonal diagnosis. This was new to you and let you believe your treatment might become less humiliating. Your medicine dosage was gradually reduced, and some of the unpleasant visible side-effects moderated. You got your period, which you hadn't had in 11 years, as menstrual cessation is a side-effect of antipsychotics.

One day in April 2004 I witnessed one consequence of Luise's not working through her traumas. Staff on the ward at St. Hans phoned, asking me to come. They couldn't understand what had happened to her. She was as scared as a hunted animal, and the staff couldn't get through to her. She fought and raved, shouting 'No, I won't.' Thank goodness she calmed down a little when I arrived. I told the staff that the ward she'd just moved to was the same place where she got drug poisoning in 1992-1994, where she'd been strapped down and subjected to forced injections, and where her bedding caught fire. The old traumas that she'd buried had resurfaced when she saw this place again.

Your good psychiatrist took you seriously and arranged conferences with the psychologist. You were really happy about this.

You would never miss a conference, no matter how tired or ill you were.

How wonderful it was to see you starting to get some of your energy back. You began to talk again about traveling. You began to follow what was happening in the city's cultural milieu. One thing you wanted to see was the exhibition of the English painter Turner's landscapes. We had earlier seen his paintings in London.

On September 23, 2004, you were discharged from St. Hans Hospital.

The discharge letter says in part:
'During hospitalization we found no evidence of mental retardation. The patient appears of normal intelligence, well-oriented, and can problem-solve ... The patient's medication has included Seroquel in relatively high doses (1200 mg daily dose in combination with a high dose of Orap). Our experience is that the patient is treatment-resistant to the medication. Treatment with antipsychotics has been reduced because of side-effects, e.g. has resumed menstruation. She has been started on birth control pills, partly to reduce the risk of osteoporosis ... The patient no longer has extrapyramidal side-effects (strange involuntary movements), but there is still a mild form of tardive dyskinesia (involuntary grimacing) ... The immediate plan is that no medication changes should be made for the next one to two years, since the patient should be regarded as treatment-resistant. It can then be assessed whether the patient's medication should gradually be further reduced. The patient was examined because of her vomiting.'

You finally took the tests they had earlier refused that show how medication is absorbed by CYP enzymes. It was no surprise to me that you did have a significantly lower metabolization rate than normal.

Now that your drug intake had been significantly reduced, you had renewed hope that better times lay ahead. Since you'd had your good psychiatrist for only six months, there was a limit to how much she could reduce your medication, since it is too dangerous to go too fast after so many years of treatment.

33

RETURN TO HELL

'Aha! Here is a subject,' exclaimed the king
when he saw the little prince coming.
The little prince asked himself: 'How can he recognize me
when he had never seen me before?'
He did not know how the world is simplified for kings.
To them all men are subjects.

Antoine de Saint-Exupéry *The Little Prince*

After returning from the psychiatric hospital to the Sundbygård care home, you went through a bad period. Your drug intake was sharply reduced, and this had consequences. Disorder is created in the brain's neurotransmitter system after significant changes in medication. But you just had to get through it, and your care-giver was a great support for you during this period. I guessed it would take three weeks before the chaos in your head would fade away. But it actually took only two weeks. Then you entered the usual vomiting phase, which surprised neither me nor the staff, because even though you were taking significantly less medicine it was still far above your tolerance level.

You became more and more clear-headed. And you began to re-turn to your old self – interested in your surroundings, full of zest for life. It was wonderful to see.

Sofus convened a follow-up conference to discuss Luise's 18-month stay at St. Hans Psychiatric Hospital. My companion Charlotte and I had plenty of ammunition. My goal was to come up with a long-term treatment plan where Luise's drug intake could be further reduced after one to two years, in accordance with St. Hans Hospital's evaluation, which I trusted. I naturally also discussed Luise's worrisome tendency to constantly throw up.

The written record of the conference on November 8, 2004 states:
'... Unfortunately, the mother expects that a reduction in medication should be considered. This is somewhat contrary to my position ... Regarding somatic matters, the patient's mother states the patient has had vomiting fits for many years. I cannot remember this.'

It was incomprehensible to me that Sofus, Luise's assigned psychiatrist, could not remember anything about the vomiting. He himself had mentioned the problem in all her previous chart notes and sent her for countless unpleasant gastrointestinal examinations on the same grounds. And now he could not remember anything about it!

The staff had asked to meet with Sofus because you were throwing up so much. The meeting took place on November 19. I stood outside and waited. I had delivered a letter to Sofus about the problem before the meeting. Your main caregiver, Dorte, who was present at the meeting, told me afterwards that you led the discussion yourself, and that she'd never seen you so strong and focused as in this conference. Dorte said she had backed you up by saying: 'Luise felt better and was more clear-headed than I've ever seen her before – a hundred percent.' The record of the meeting does not even indicate that your caregiver was present.

The record states:
'The patient says that she must stick a finger down her throat to induce vomiting. In addition, the patient is very talkative, digressive and somewhat disconnected. Reports there are several people inside her room who are friendly, having a hard time and homeless. They are friendly but do not talk to her because they are invisible ... I *(i.e. Sofus)* ask about her orientation: The patient does not know what day of the

week it is. When asked about the month, she replies the month before December, when Christmas is. I ask what year it is, and get no reply...'

What Sofus wrote about your lack of orientation is not true. If anyone knew the date, it was you. You even had an engagement calendar I'd given you as a present. You had memorized my entire schedule with your remarkable memory. You knew when we had scheduled get-togethers, knew the dates for upcoming exhibitions and how long they were running. You often called me to suggest I avoid driving home the next day at 8 pm, when the soccer crowd would be leaving the park and jamming up our neighborhood.

After Luise was tested at St. Hans Hospital, they had rejected the 'mentally retarded' diagnosis. So why is Sofus making Luise out to be mentally retarded? Lack of orientation about time and place is one of the criteria for making this diagnosis. Her caregiver said quite specifically that Luise had been very clear-headed and focused. I do not understand this.

The next family conference took place on December 13. Charlotte again sat by me. Luise's good caregiver, Dorte, took the floor and described how the staff perceived Luise. Among other things, she said they felt Luise behaved very differently from other residents diagnosed with schizophrenia. She stressed that the group is, of course, very varied, but it was as if Luise was a complete outsider – I have often heard the same from day staff on the various wards where Luise stayed over the years. She discussed the problem of Luise's throwing up, reporting that the care team had talked about how much better Luise felt after prolonged vomiting. Sofus said that regardless of whether the diagnosis was right or wrong, it could never be erased. It was a very long meeting, in which Dorte argued well for the staff's position. At the meeting we asked to see the record of Luise's conference with Sofus on November 19.

I was shocked to see Sofus's record stating: 'Urgent call from Sundbygård staff. The patient has been increasingly psychotic recently and has been vomiting. If the patient does not improve, she should be hospitalized.' This was not at all correct, so Dorte brought out the chart and started to recite from the staff's daily patient notes, which indicated Luise had been very sociable and happy. She had helped with the daily chores. She had not received any additional medication, as she normally did. Therefore there was no evidence of 'increasing psychosis.' I asked how it was possible to observe increasing psychosis at a single meeting – if it were increasing, it would be happening gradually. Sofus said he had met Luise in the hallway and saw that she seemed psychotic.

Why did Sofus write that Luise was increasingly psychotic when she was feeling better than she had in a long time? I was very worried when I saw the chart note. Was he perhaps setting up Luise for an imminent increase in her medication? An observation of increasing psychosis usually resulted in more medication.

Luise had now been at St. Hans Hospital for 18 months. The reason for her being there was to stabilize her and adjust her medication. Her dose had been adjusted and reduced considerably. She was feeling better, and now it looked to me as if everything was about to fall flat. I did not understand his motives.

The minutes of this meeting included a great deal about the World Health Organization's diagnostic indications for schizophrenia and a little about Dorte's and the staff's views on Luise's diagnosis. It was all written rather vaguely, but there it was. Several people saw this record. I got access to it two weeks later, only to discover a whole new version of the record. The key passage – 'Urgent call from Sundbygård staff. The patient has been increasingly psychotic recently and has been vomiting. If the patient does not improve, she should be hospitalized.' – was deleted.

The minutes of the family conference on December 13 now only dealt with Luise's vomiting. Now it resembled the letter I had delivered by hand on November 19, though flavored with the usual assertion that my concerns were clearly unjustified. The sentence I wrote predicting that Luise would be hospitalized within a month if things went as usual was not included.

34

EVEN MORE MEDICATION

What lies behind these stunningly bad treatment outcomes?
A basic cause is that psychiatrists have apparently forgotten
that they're treating real live people. They only see patients
as individuals whose brain chemistry is out of order.

Herluf Dalhoff, specialist in general medicine,
***Kristeligt Dagblad* newspaper**

Mental health care is not producing good treatment results despite, or perhaps precisely because of, the fact that antipsychotic drug doses have risen dramatically. The Danish Pharmacy Association's 2007 report puts the increase at around 24% between 2002 and 2006. More and more patients are suffering from the severe, long-term side effects of antipsychotics, and these drugs are a contributory factor in the considerably shortened longevity of this population group. The number of judicial treatment sentences is constantly increasing. The number of young people in mental health treatment on Social Security disability is increasing year by year.

I will briefly try to illustrate why things often go awry, along with a few suggestions on how things could be improved.

Just to be clear, I do not question that people suffering from acute psychosis and in deep distress must receive all the medication necessary to ease their suffering. Dosages should simply be reduced when the psychosis has subsided, and then conferences with a psychologist offered so the patient gets treatment for the underlying cause of the psychotic outbreak. I am not questioning the use of psychotropic drugs. What I see as the problem is that a very large group of people is treated with massive doses of medication for years on end. They are categorized as 'chroni-cally ill patients' and are often treated negligently. They do not undergo the required examinations and their drug side-effects are not evaluated, as required by law. It does not occur to the specialists that, despite the heavy medication, their patients do not improve and in many cases get worse. No attention is paid to the fact that they suffer from dangerous and destructive side-effects that make their lives unnecessarily difficult and squalid.

They are abandoned, and the inappropriate treatment of this large group continues, unnoticed by the people responsible.

The Board of Health is the body that oversees medical treatment in Denmark. They need to sharpen their control and oversight of psy-chotropic drug prescribing. This can be done through a patient's digital medication profile. It is also their job to check that doctors follow the guidelines laid down for the evaluation and monitoring of side-effects – and give a reprimand for non-compliance.

The Board takes no action, although it is clear from the studies – undertaken by themselves, among others – that their guidelines are not followed. Medication is overused. The compulsory evaluations and monitoring are rarely carried out.

Research Director Professor Birte Glenthøj:
'It is important to remember that if medication does not help, it does not necessarily mean the patient is receiving too little, as it could easily be because the dose is too high ... Because of potentially serious side-effects, such as movement disorders or increased risk of cardiovascular disease, it is also very important to constantly weigh the beneficial effects of treatment against possible side-effects.'
Dagens Medicin (Today's Medicine)

The Danish Regions interest group wrote in March 2009: 'We must have world-class psychiatry.' Eight visions are listed for achieving this

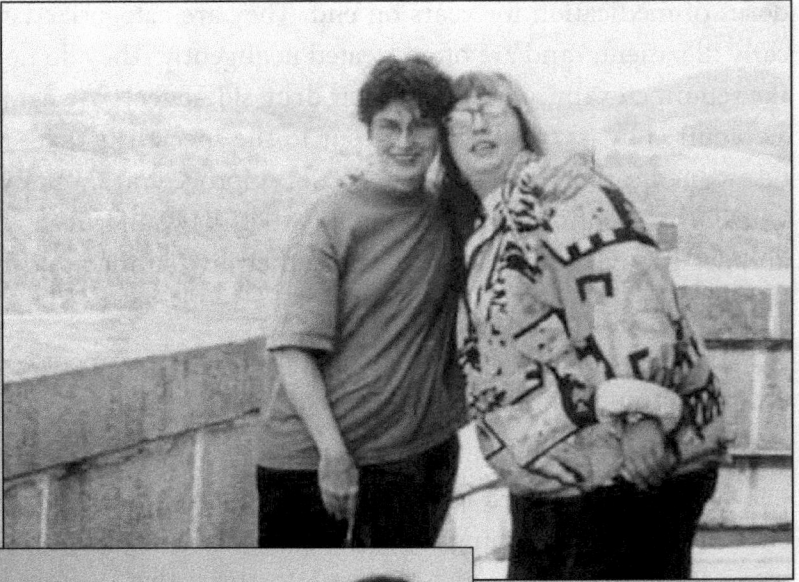

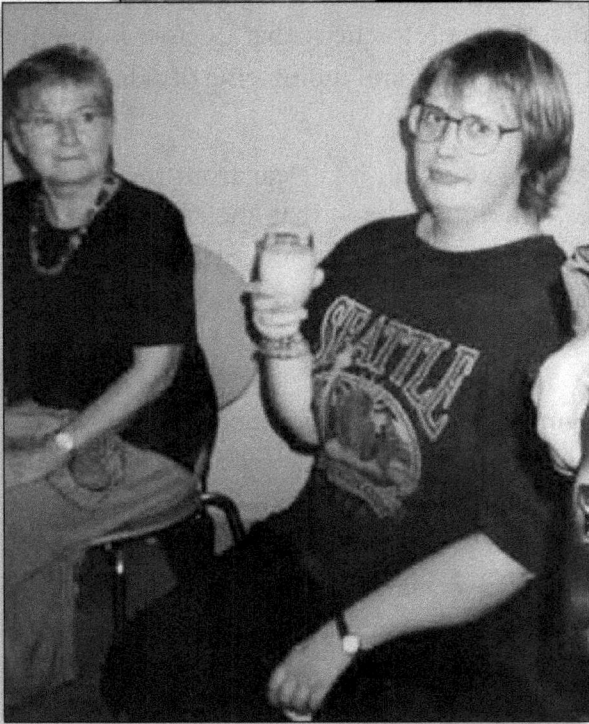

*With Marsha in the
Columbia Gorge,
Oregon (top); and
at a birthday party.*

goal. One of them is: 'We will reduce the excessive mortality among people with mental illness.'

In my opinion, we'll never get world-class psychiatry as long as the practitioner culture is stuck in the mind-set that psychiatric patients' problems are caused solely by improper brain chemistry, which can only be remedied by drugs. This biological approach is destructive and mechanical. Medication obviously cannot stand alone. We forget that this is all about vulnerable people who, like everyone else, need recognition and hope so they can get on with their lives. They need to talk to professionals about their problems. Unfortunately, there's not much opportunity for that in Denmark today.

A patient chart is a document that follows a person for life. It is important that it provide an all-encompassing picture. Currently this does not happen. Permeating most charts is an assumption that treatment is about medication. The chart often resembles a summary of a series of snapshots/consultations, each describing how the patient feels here and now and what drugs they are taking or should take. The diagnosis is depicted, not the person it applies to. More often than not, the chart even fails to note the patient's treatment history.

Then there's the issue of false information in chart notes. This is usually impossible to substantiate. It is relatively rare that staff, family and friends get to see the record soon after the conferences they attend. But how often do we hear people in treatment or next of kin saying that what is written in the record is, in their view, distorted or completely incorrect?

I have a few suggestions for avoiding incorrect and sometimes fatal information in such an important document.

Psychiatrist and patient should look at the draft minutes together after a conference. If there is disagreement over the formulation, there should be discussion about the differing perceptions. The same procedure should be followed after a conference with next of kin.

This would require a lot more dialogue, a doctor-patient interaction on equal footing. And it seems the Danish mental health system is not set up for this today. But it has to happen sooner or later.

I think it should also be possible to get a second opinion on both diagnosis and treatment. This is normal within other specialist areas. My reasoning behind this is that the only metric for making a psychiatric diagnosis is the physician's evaluation, often based on no more than a snapshot of the patient. The same goes for medication.

Over the years I have written to several leading psychiatrists asking if they could support me with a thorough evaluation. They could only refer me back to Luise's psychiatrist.

However, I finally found a psychiatrist who would talk to me about Luise's diagnosis and treatment. His evaluation was based on what I told him about her psychological tests at the Institute of Psychology, which indicated she suffered from Asperger's syndrome. He said he would contact Luise's psychiatrist and was sure that the two of them together could devise a long-term drug discontinuation plan for Luise. I think he said it would take over five years, because people with this diagnosis are very sensitive to antipsychotic medication and might be harmed by the treatment. A month later the doctor phoned to inform me that Luise's psychiatrist refused to cooperate. I remember I cried into the phone on hearing this and said I might just as well wait for Luise to die.

That came to pass four days later.

From my experience and that of many others, it is clear that psychiatrists do not find it necessary to consult with others about their patients. This was more or less what Sofus indicated in his letter, after I asked for a second opinion. So I don't see any other solution to the problem of these patients, who drag themselves through life in an unnecessary neuroleptic straitjacket, than that the Board of Health follow their own program and make sure their guidelines are being observed – and act on any contraventions.

35

COMMOTION IN THE WARD

By calling another human being 'mentally ill'
we place that person outside
a meaningful human world,
perceived as 'object' rather than 'subject.'

Medical Director Finn Jørgensen

'Commotion in the ward.' This was the only thing they could say about your best friend Suzanne's sudden death. The beginning of January 2005 would show that things could get worse than I could ever have dreamt in my wildest nightmares.

Luise was admitted to the psychiatric ward at Amager Hospital in early January. I had anticipated this and had written to Sofus on November 22 to inform him.

The reason was the same as for previous admissions.

She had been throwing up for five weeks. This stopped in early December, after which the usual thing happened, namely once she started keeping down her medication, it affected her like a drug overdose.

At Amager Hospital they immediately increased her medication dose significantly.

Sofus took an active part in increasing Luise's drug intake, despite the fact that he had been involved in the discharge conference at St. Hans Psychiatric Hospital some three months earlier. Here it was explained that a year and a half of observation and several medication increases and decreases led to the conclusion that Luise should take as little anti-psychotic medication as possible.

Luise, why do you think the psychiatrist was acting contrary to St. Hans Hospital's recommendations? The argument for you being hospitalized, totally against your will, was precisely to get your medication adjusted. Your medicine was adjusted to around half of what you were taking before being admitted. Why let the doctor who arranged this hospital transfer again increase your drug dose shortly after your return home? After all, this is what made your 18-month hospital stay therapeutically futile!

Luise, over the years you had a lot of trouble with side-effects. No one could doubt this. Even your psychiatrists couldn't miss your strange involuntary movements and grimaces and your agitated state. When you did complain about the side-effects, you were promptly told: 'You have to choose between plague and cholera.'

The medical journals frequently point out that psychiatrists should be aware of the side-effects of antipsychotic drugs, advising that problems can often be resolved by a dosage reduction. The Danish Psychiatric Society's guidelines for treatment with antipsychotics (1998) emphasize this point: 'The side-effects of antipsychotic drugs sometimes counteract their therapeutic effect and lead to new psychological symptoms.'

The increased medication you received after admission to Amager Hospital on January 3, 2005, made you worse – which was no surprise to us. The worst part was that this time you lost faith that you could ever get out of drug hell. My heart sank when on one of my visits you limply asked me: 'Mom, do you think it's better in heaven?' I can't remember how I answered this pitiable question.

But I was in no doubt about the reason for your question.

I heard less and less of your delightful laughter. It became increasingly difficult for you to engage with the world around you.

However, when I told you about my upcoming study tour to Egypt, I could see your sad eyes light up a little.

I was leaving for Egypt on January 20, where I planned to stay at Agatha Christie's Cataract Hotel at Aswan. This is what cheered you up a little.

Two years earlier we had been to the Moesgaard Museum near Aarhus, Denmark's second city.

We were on one of our 'musical holidays' at your uncle Mogens' place. That's what you always called our stays with Mogens, because he gave you unconditional permission to play anything from his vast CD collection. It was pure heaven for you to sit in front of those stacks of CDs. You and Mogens had the same taste in music.

At Moesgaard there was a small exhibition about Agatha Christie's life as a writer, with visual aids to guide us through some of her books.

The first exhibit we saw was a scale model of the train from Paddington Station in London. One of Agatha Christie's detective novels is called '4.50 from Paddington.' This transported us both to dreamland. We'd often taken the train from Paddington Station, heading for our hideaway in Cornwall at Jenni and Dziga's place – and their cat Spider, who always slept with you when we were visiting.

We actually once took the train from Paddington around 4.50 pm, though without witnessing a murder. We had a good laugh over that. You of course had a funny comment about the Paddington train: 'Mom, even though I might have tried to get rid of you on the train to Cornwall, it wouldn't have been possible, because the carriages don't have compartments any more!' And then you broke out in your lovely gurgling laughter.

There was also a reconstruction of the Orient Express, which would lead me to the novel 'Murder on the Orient Express.'

We saw the Nile steamer where 'Death on the Nile' unfolds. Near the Nile steamer we saw Agatha Christie's suite at the old

Cataract Hotel, the hotel where I was hoping to stay. Agatha Christie lived there for long periods and several of her novels were written there.

At the Moesgaard exhibition we decided we had to travel to Aswan at some point and stay at this hotel. Of course we would also sail on the Nile.

It was a wonderful trip to look forward to, and our dreams and fantasies were stretched to unimaginable dimensions.

We agreed that while on my study tour I would start planning our trip to Egypt. We imagined it would happen in autumn 2005. Summer is too hot in these parts. Susanne, your friend at the care home was staying in the room next door. She was also excited about our Egypt plans.

I visited you on January 19 to say goodbye, and you said you were looking forward to my coming home so you could hear all about Egypt. I promised to buy a scarab for you. To the Egyptians the scarab is a sign of rebirth and eternal life.

Suzanne also wished me bon voyage and I promised her a scarab, too.

I phoned from the airport at 8.05 am the next day to say goodbye.

But we couldn't even talk, because of loud terrified screaming coming from nearby in the ward.

The screaming continued, and you were totally paralyzed and unable to say anything on the phone.

You hung up without saying goodbye.

I arrived home the evening of January 27.

Calling from the airport, I chattered on about Agatha Christie's hotel, the boat trip on the Nile and the scarab.

You sounded dejected and uninterested.

You had little interest in talking, so we agreed I should visit you the following day.

The next day I learned the reason for your despondency.

The scream I'd heard when I phoned from the airport happened when Suzanne collapsed on the floor.

She died within minutes.

You were deeply unhappy and still in shock when I came to visit.

All you said was: 'I'll be next.'

You were completely shattered.

You didn't want to hear about Egypt. You didn't want the scarab, because you now believed it wouldn't help.

The day before I left you said you were so much looking forward to my coming home, so I could tell you all about Egypt.

Now I was home, you were no longer interested in making plans to travel there.

Dreams of the Nile, the Cataract Hotel and Agatha Christie were irrelevant now.

You talked about Susanne but still would rather not get into the subject. You seemed empty.

Your friend had fallen. Perhaps even before your eyes?

I still don't know, because you never talked about it.

I know only that you repeated desperately, 'I'll be the next to die.'

I told the care staff on the ward that they should realize this was your best friend who had died and you definitely needed to talk about this traumatic event.

The staff's response was that you had not been affected by Susanne's death.

So where was the staff's psychological insight?

Of course you were deeply affected, but you may not have been able to articulate your feelings when you 'had the chance' right after it happened.

The staff told me they had gathered all the patients together right after Suzanne's death, but you appeared completely untouched by this shocking event.

This left me speechless.

Your apparent calmness obviously reflected your state of shock. But the staff chose to interpret your lack of response as indifference.

This was how they could justify to themselves and others that there was no reason to comfort you or talk to you about what had occurred, because 'you were totally indifferent.'

Luise, you often said that the hospital personnel never treated patients as people with normal feelings. Their handling of Susanne's death, as it related to the rest of you, told me you were right.

If a person in the normal world unexpectedly dropped dead in a workplace or a schoolyard, an employer or school principal would immediately call in a psychologist to help deal with the crisis. The expert would understand that witnesses to the death might have various response patterns that amounted to post-traumatic shock symptoms, which would need to be worked through.

If you find yourself inside the walls of a psychiatric ward, the staff can just disappear into their cubicles and pretend nothing happened. With their 'good education' in psychiatry, they see that all the patients are completely unaffected when one of their fellow-patients collapses and dies.

On January 20, that fatal day when Susanne died, the staff wrote this about you in the nursing record: 'Rather troubled because of the commotion in the ward this morning. Seems everything is wrong with her and she's asking us to take her blood pressure.'

This was the only thing ever written about your reaction. You got lots of extra sedation, so much, in fact, that the next day, according to the nursing record, you staggered around and often looked like you were about to fall. But again this was simply interpreted as posturing.

36

DISEMPOWERMENT

*The treatment of the mentally ill through the ages
has been marked by human stupidity, ignorance and cynicism,
without regard to the fact that treatment methods were often
directly harmful and not unlike torture. This is true even today.
But ignorance is no excuse today. We, the people of Denmark,
must now demand that our politicians conduct
a thorough review of treatment practices.*

**Herluf Dalhoff, specialist in general medicine,
Kristeligt Dagblad newspaper**

Do care providers believe that coercion and disempowerment can help psychiatric patients get better? I don't know. But Luise had been broken. She became more and more exasperated, shut inside herself.

After reading the chart notes, I realize that coercion, both overt and covert, plays a much greater role in 'treatment' than I ever had imagined.

Initially Luise fought back, which resulted in long-term coercive measures. I can see that eventually just the threat of forcible measures was enough to make Luise simply give in.

Luise, according to your chart, you yourself on several occasions asked to be strapped down. You preferred this vile coercive measure to the even worse alternative: extra medication and/or drugs by injection. You had wide experience of the terrifying consequences.

The chart note dated June 30, 2005, when you were strapped down and injected with Valium plus a dose of Cisordinol, illustrates this: 'The patient comes into the staff room and says she feels bad. She slips to the floor and for the next ten minutes suffers several very brief fits, lying on her back and hitting her arms and legs on the floor with rapid movements.' Similar fits were previously recorded in the chart.

You would think that talking might be a normal part of treatment on a psychiatric ward, but this wasn't the case for you, Luise. A chat with your doctor would have given you the chance to tell how you felt about your treatment, and why you were afraid of the antipsychotic medication. It would also have helped you to process the terrifying experience it must have been to suffer drug poisoning.

It was amazing how much better Luise felt when the doctor at St. Hans Psychiatric Hospital listened to her. And things got even better in her sessions there with a psychologist.

The 'help' Luise got after Suzanne's death (so much medication that she staggered around) tells me that the lack of reaction from the other patients in the ward was also due to fear.

Although they were left to deal with the shock, the screams and, worst of all, the fear that they might be next to die from overmedication, they made every effort not to react emotionally to the situation.

People hospitalized in a psychiatric ward know that the treatment offered for an intense reaction is rarely soothing conversation, but rather the restraints, possibly supplemented with a syringe.

The Icelandic psychiatrist Petur Hauksson, who chaired the Council of Europe's Committee against Torture, was quoted in the daily newspaper *Politiken* in October 2002, saying of Danish psychiatry: 'It seemed as if strapping patients down was part of normal psychiatric practice. As if it had become part of the tradition.'

When the committee again visited Denmark in 2004, they noted there had been no reduction at all in these coercive measures – indeed, quite the contrary.

How many friends and family members have visited a psychiatric ward and seen one of the caregiver team sitting in a chair, knitting or reading outside a locked door?

Patients knew that behind that door was a fellow-patient strapped down and completely alone. As visitors, we didn't always know this.

The person outside the door sat there in case the restrained patient started to yell, in which case they would be sedated with an injection. The guard at the door also had to make sure the patient did not get seriously ill while strapped down. Sitting by the door was a security measure, not a routine intended to ease the patient's pain.

Extra pills or injections for a patient who is depressed or scared, rather than conversation, seems to have become a part of the Danish psychiatric tradition.

The following is extracted from an article that appeared in *Politiken* in November 2005, four months after Luise's death: 'For the first time in years the practice of strapping patients in restraints has decreased significantly, according to figures from the National Board of Health. In other words, we're starting to talk to patients. This lets patients feel they are being met face to face, are respected and are in good hands. It creates confidence and a sense of shared responsibility, and we realize patients can take much more responsibility than we had assumed.'

Under the heading 'Restraints can be avoided,' *Politiken* wrote on January 13, 2006:

'It costs almost nothing, and it works. At the 22 psychiatric wards in Denmark staff have reduced the use of coercive measures by talking with patients ... These positive outcomes have led the Health Minister to require that the new law governing psychiatric practice should include a provision to closely monitor restrained patients, and that staff be required to talk with patients after such a coercive measure is used.'

I think we should have a law requiring that staff on psychiatric wards must talk with their patients in general, not just when they have been strapped down.

If you visit Amager Hospital psychiatric ward's website, you will see: 'Offering hospital care based on the integration of biological, psychological and social-psychiatric treatment modes. The goal is individual treatment tailored to each patient's needs and resources.'

I don't recognize this from Luise's stay there. I heard a similar description from a psychologist from a metropolitan area hospital at a meeting of the national association Mind. The meeting was headlined 'Daily life in a psychiatric ward.'

When the speaker was finished, there was time for an hour's debate.

The first comment came from a former patient. His picturesque description of therapy treatment in the wards he had frequented struck a familiar chord.

He described it as follows: 'There are a lot of doped-up people in a lounge. They all sit in their chairs, deep in their own thoughts and shut off from the outside world. They smoke one cigarette after another. Not a word is uttered in the room, unless a patient runs out of cigarettes and asks: Does anyone have a cigarette to spare?

The person gets a cigarette, and the deep silence resumes. At five o'clock one of the caregiver team shows up. Now patients have to agree who should set the table, and who should carry the food in, and so on. It's called DLA training. Here, patients 'learn' daily living activities, like setting the table and doing what's necessary to serve dinner.'

No one else had any comments.

Back to January 20, 2005, when you, Luise, gave up all hope because your friend had died and you were sure you would be next. It was also the day the staff didn't believe it was important to talk to you about your fears and your sorrows, but instead gave you generous doses of extra medication.

From the day on it was hard to make you happy.

Just as bad was the fact that I had lost faith that your treatment would ever improve.

37

DESTINY CALLS

*I find myself in a universe of shock, where nothing mattered.
The voice might just as well have said
that a plane had crashed in our neighborhood
or that war had broken out.
Nothing really mattered. I just wanted some peace.*

The phone rang on July 15 at 6:30 in the morning.

It wasn't you calling. A calm, cool female voice from Amager Hospital asked if I was the mother of Luise Hjerming Christensen.

The strange thing is I'd been expecting this phone call for several years.

I'd had so many nightmares and crystal-clear dreams about your death. In many ways I felt almost prepared.

However, along with the fear I'd always had hope. Hope that you would find a psychiatrist who could see that your treatment was wrong and who would dare to insist on making changes, so you could eventually be taken off the strong medication.

Hope and love were my driving force.

The woman then said, 'I have to tell you I just got a call from intensive care unit C2, saying that the person on watch outside the room next to Luise's suddenly heard a thud from inside Luise's room. He goes in and finds Luise lying convulsed on the floor. His back-up arrives and administers CPR.'

The voice continued, and I screamed: 'No, no, no!' She said 'Yes' and droned on, but now I was screaming so wildly I couldn't even hear what she said. I could only hear this quiet voice humming in the background, like muzak in a supermarket.

I screamed: 'Is she dead?'

'Yes.'

I shouted, 'No, no, no, it can't be. You've killed her with your medicine. That's what I always said. You were going to kill her.'

Now I couldn't even make out the words spoken by this calm voice that just kept on babbling.

Then the voice became more insistent: 'Dorrit, Dorrit, just try to listen. As soon as you calm down, would you like to come here and see her?' I wept in total despair, as the calm, ice-cold voice echoed eerily in the background.

'How fast can you get over here?'

I was in a universe of shock.

A universe where nothing mattered any more. The voice might as well have said that a plane had crashed in our neighborhood, or that war had broken out.

Nothing really mattered. I just wanted some peace.

Leave me alone.

The monotone voice calmly droned on, now insisting: 'Dorrit, Dorrit, if you come in, we can talk about it.'

'Talk about it.' She made it sound like there had been some slight hitch in the workplace, a minor misunderstanding we could set to rights by talking.

What was there to talk about? I'd just received final notification of my daughter's death.

I immediately called my sister, Elsebeth, who was on vacation north of Copenhagen.

She also froze with shock but would of course come as quickly as possible.

Then I called my friend Vibeke, who lives nearby.

Before Vibeke arrived I got another call from the hospital.

This time the cold female voice said that if we wanted to have flowers on Luise's deathbed we had to bring them ourselves!

I called Vibeke again and told her about the new problem over flowers. Not that it was a problem to find them, as we live in an area with flowers everywhere. But in my state of shock my big problem was that I had to have red roses but had no rosebush clippers.

All this unfolded in slow motion.

Vibeke brought garden shears and garden gloves, and we rushed out and cut a huge bunch of roses. A total panic reaction from both of us.

In the end, how much could it matter whether Luise got roses for her brief stay in the hospital morgue?

She was dead! There was no way around this.

Around eight o'clock I got a third call from Amager Hospital.

Now the voice said: 'If you want to see Luise before she's taken away, you have to come now.'

I yelled back tearfully: 'I can't just come out there alone to see you people, who have killed her, and say my final farewell to Luise, the person in my life I love the most! Do you want me to jump on my bike or take the subway right after my daughter has died?'

The voice suggested I could take a taxi. But somehow I couldn't relate to this. I always took the subway or rode the bike when I visited her, so these two modes of transport were the only ones that made sense to me.

The voice kept insisting: 'It's important that you come here now if you want to see Luise. We can also offer you a doctor conference when you get here. Are you interested?' I must have answered yes.

Luckily, Elsebeth soon arrived. We drove out to Amager Hospital to say a last goodbye to Luise.

Two well-prepared doctors were there when Elsebeth and I arrived at the unit.

We were first shown into the room where you lay. The caregivers from your ward never made an appearance. There was a nurse we didn't know sitting by your bed. She seemed to radiate empathy. I think she even expressed her condolences.

Luise, this was the sole glimmer of compassion we felt on this final heartrending visit.

Otherwise, all we got was aggressive bureaucratic posturing.

The sight that greeted me on that fatal Friday morning, when I saw you, my beloved Luise, lying dead in the white sheets, did nothing to allay my grief. I'd always heard that when people were dead they looked peaceful, and this usually gave next of kin some consolation to see a loved one had found peace.

You did not look peaceful.

You had the usual angst-ridden wrinkle between your eyes.

You were blue in the face, with blue-violet lips.

The profusion of red roses we'd hurriedly plucked an hour earlier to put on your shroud only highlighted that blue, anguished look.

I'd picked red roses because you associated them with love, and you always brought red roses for everyone you loved. Yet red roses seemed all wrong this morning.

I've always been able to control my thoughts and feelings in public.

I've practiced for years to look as though I have perfect control over my life.

I've always felt that a single mother is expected to be in control, with a firm grip on any situation. You don't just fall to pieces and get all theatrical – that's a sign of weakness and incompetence.

I was not prepared for this.

All those years of learned self-control was wiped out in one second.

38

'An unintended event'

A patient chart consists of organized records,
which include details of the patient's condition,
examinations conducted and planned, and
treatment, including what information
is presented to and received from the patient.

Regulation 846 governing doctors' record-keeping duties

Your death was described as 'an unintended event' by the doctor in the intensive care unit.

He was the one who had ordered the injection. At his side sat your regular consultant psychiatrist who was supposed to follow you while you were 'temporarily' admitted to the ward.

There was no offer of condolences.

The doctors seemed angry, dismissive and insensitive.

Elsebeth asked why they had not listened to my warnings.

A week earlier I'd told them that more drugs – and especially prolonged-release medication – would be your death, because you couldn't throw them up. My argument against increased medication six days earlier had been that no psychiatrist knew exactly how much medication you could actually tolerate, since you always vomited.

Luise, I really did everything in my power to stop them giving you prolonged-release medication.

The answer to Elsebeth's question was: 'We went by the book.'

In the fog of my shocked state I was almost transported into the religious domain.

Was it the Bible or the Koran they were alluding to?

Both these holy books are referred to as the book.

I don't think the doctor was talking about holy books.

But one thing is for sure – you didn't fit the book, Luise.

In any case, they had not acted by the book. Luise was given a new antipsychotic drug on top of the three she was already taking. This contravenes the Board of Health guideline that says two drugs at a time can be administered in exceptional cases, but as far as possible doctors should avoid giving more than one.

There is nothing in the record that shows what information Luise was given on prolonged release injections, or what she said about it. There should have been.

The only thing written about this heavy medication increase is as follows: July 8, 2005: 'Today talked with the patient. She wants medicine to keep the voices away, but she does not want an injection. I tell her I intend to propose prolonged-release treatment for an extended period. The patient became seriously agitated. She yells and screams and slams her fist hard on the table, but quickly calms down and apologizes for her behavior.'

On July 14: 'The patient was persuaded today to take prolonged-release medicine.' Then a few words about the dose and about her feeling well.

That is all that is noted in the chart about such an important decision.

The sentence 'The patient was persuaded today to take prolonged-release medicine' is ominous.

The autopsy also revealed marks around her body, which the coroner could not explain. I have no doubt these stem from what happened when she got the injection.

I had called Luise the afternoon of July 14. She was angry and did not want me to visit. This worried me.

I then phoned the ward and was told that she was doing fine and she just did not want a visit from me. When I asked if there had been a change in her medication – I dreaded the injection the doctor had talked about, which I said would be her death – they replied they had decided to inform me about any medication changes only once a week, so I could find out about this the following Thursday. Now I got really scared.

The next morning at 6.30 am I got the phone call telling me Luise was dead.

I can see from the medication record that Luise had already been injected when I phoned her. There is nothing in the record about the injection, except the time.

Medical law requires that a patient's chart must record what information the patient has received about a new product and what the patient has articulated about it. Nothing is noted.

It was perhaps understandable that none of the caregiver team came to express condolences. Around 9:30 am the ward was usually swarming with people, but everyone was gone when we arrived.

Elsebeth then asked why they had not accepted St. Hans Hospital's view that you were drug-resistant, which according to our information meant there was no reason to administer excessive doses. I cannot remember the answer to that question.

Your death was described as 'an unintended event.'

For you and for me it was the most wretched and definitive thing that could possibly happen.

Your life was cut short in an instant. I was deprived of the most precious thing in my life in an instant.

Why couldn't I help you? Why wouldn't any psychiatrist listen to you or me? The psychiatrists all knew better. This meant your death.

Luise shines no more.
I cannot find the words.
I am left with
a crushing grief.
Luise was sacrificed
at the grim altar of absurdity.

Antipsychotic drugs are not candy.

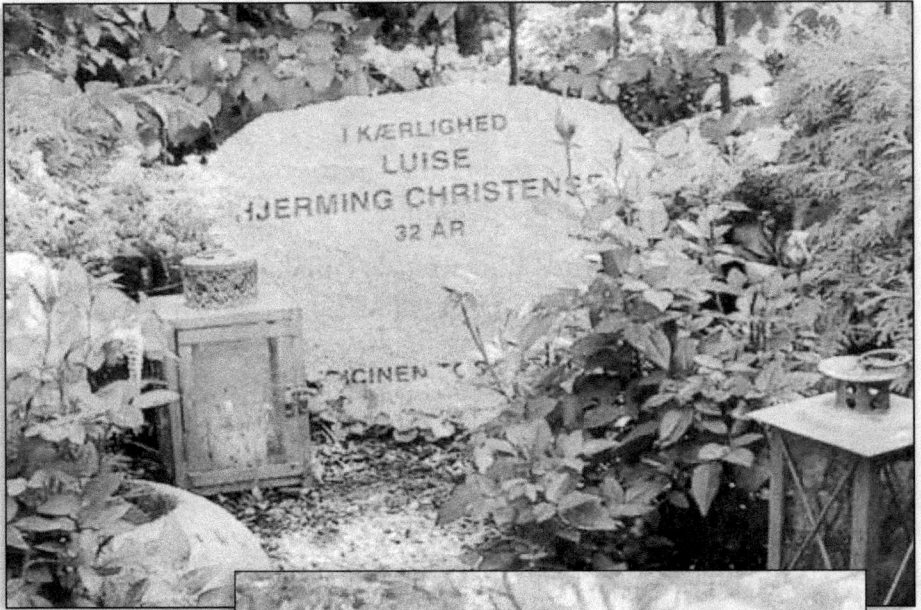

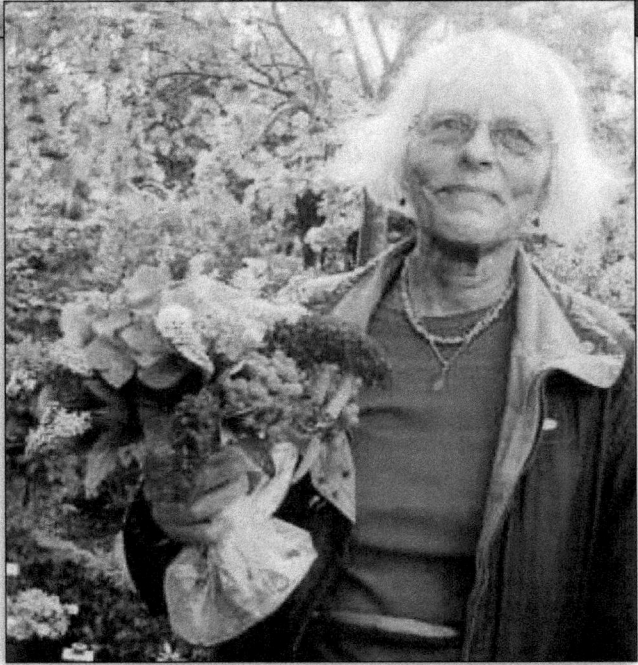

Luise's gravestone in Copenhagen.
The inscription reads: 'The medicine took my life.'

Epilogue

Fighting the system

They all said to me: 'Don't bother filing a complaint. It's a degrading and exhausting process. And you'll never get anywhere with it. Psychiatrists are as thick as thieves.'

Of course, I had to complain. It should have been obvious that Luise died because she got too much medication. She suddenly collapsed and could not be resuscitated. According to the autopsy report, she had no previously undetected diseases. She had been given far more than the recommended dose of four antipsychotics and two different tranquilizers – as a rule a patient should be given only one antipsychotic. I was confident the conclusion would be that Luise's treatment was not up to standard.

I reported Luise's death to the police, the Patient Complaints Commission and the Patient Insurance Association soon after she died. Surely there was at least the possibility of a negligent homicide investigation.

The police received my report on August 14, 2005. The only contact I had from the police was a letter dated May 19, 2006, stating they had concluded their investigation. The police did not respond when I asked whether they had received my complaint. By contrast, they had regular contact with the Copenhagen Hospital Corporation and, through them, Amager Hospital. Their first contact was on November 11, three months after I had submitted my report, when they said they found no reason to interview the doctor I had reported, but that they were awaiting the Board of Health's medical assessment of Luise's treatment.

This should have been reassuring, since the Board of Health sets guidelines for all medical treatment and is responsible for overseeing that it proceeds as prescribed.

The Board concluded that Luise had been treated in accordance with the standards of good specialist practice, which is odd because the doctor didn't even come close to following their guideline, which states: 'Monotherapy (treatment with one antipsychotic agent) with few exceptions should be the rule.'

In the wake of Luise's death, there was a running media debate about overmedication in psychiatric care and the possible consequences, or lack thereof, for doctors who do not comply with Board of Health guidelines.

The most uncompromising statements appeared in the daily newspaper *Jyllands-Posten* in March and April 2006 and in *Today's Medicine* in January 2006, where the head of the Board of Health said: 'The guidelines can, of course, be waived if there are good professional reasons for doing so. But the doctor must then be prepared that a departure from these rules may give rise to censure from the Patient Complaints Board or possibly litigation.'

Despite all the pompous statements in the media, the Board of Health expressed the opposite view in its March 9, 2006, report on Luise's treatment. Here they said that Luise had received treatment that met the standards of good specialist practice.

My complaint to the Patient Insurance Association was headlined 'Death from drug poisoning.' I named the medications Luise had been given, with special emphasis on the prolonged-release injection that she died from some ten hours after it was administered.

According to the Patient Insurance Association's psychiatry expert, Luise received the highest standard of specialist treatment. They wrote:

'1. The antipsychotic medication treatment has complied with the best professional standards. That the outcome has not been satisfactory is due to the nature of the condition and the circumstance that the profession's knowledge and treatment options are limited.

2. As stated, I believe that the risk inherent in the medication treatment must be weighed against the suffering Luise Hjerming Christensen would have undergone without treatment.'

It is incomprehensible to me that Luise's treatment was judged up to standard, when in fact they administered psychoactive pharmaceuticals that amounted to three times the highest recommended dose.

This would be like a doctor prescribing 24 Panodol tablets daily for a headache or migraine sufferer. This would be unthinkable and the doctor would immediately receive a reprimand. But why don't the same rules apply to the prescription of antipsychotic medication?

The Patient Complaints Board's decision came three years after I filed the complaint. It said that Luise had been treated in accordance with the standards of good specialist practice.

The decision took no account of public statements by leading pharmacologists from Denmark and the Nordic countries affirming that the large dose of medicine without a doubt had been the cause of Luise's sudden death.

The same doctor I had filed the complaint against was hired by the Patient Complaints Board as a psychiatric expert about six months after I filed the complaint – that is, while the case was still being considered. That told me the case got settled before it ever got started. It would simply be too inconvenient for the Board to investigate a doctor they had just hired.

One strange thing after another happened during the proceedings. Luise's death certificate said 'death from unknown causes' but as a contributory cause of death it had 'epilepsy and mental retardation.' This was false and misleading, serving only to obstruct the forensic effort to find the real cause of death. The hospital disclaimed any responsibility for these two incorrect diagnoses and said it was a matter for the police and forensic experts. I can only say that neither police nor forensic experts can tell whether a dead person is mentally retarded or epileptic. I tried to get clarification for how these diagnoses found their way to Luise's death certificate. But my efforts led nowhere.

Oddly enough, Luise's friend who had died six months earlier at the same hospital also had epilepsy listed as a contributing cause of death on her death certificate. She was not epileptic.

My complaints ultimately led nowhere, but the massive media coverage has helped launch a wide-ranging debate about the quality of mental health treatment in Denmark. This questioning shows no sign of let-up. The Board of Health has prepared several reports investigating the causes of the many sudden, unexpected deaths during treatment among people diagnosed as schizophrenics. In 2011 the Board reported that 49% of patients treated for schizophrenia are prescribed two or more anti-psychotic drugs.

My efforts to expose the deficiencies of Denmark's mental health treatment system turned into a three-year struggle. The only outcome was the system's self-congratulation for its first-class treatment of Luise.

There have unfortunately been many hundreds of 'Luise stories' in Denmark since Luise died, and they seem to be increasing year by year.

My friends were right. All my complaints ran into a brick wall.

www.ingramcontent.com/pod-product-compliance
Lightning Source LLC
Chambersburg PA
CBHW070907270326
41927CB00011B/2488